DISCOVER
SHIATSU

DISCOVER
SHIATSU

CATHERINE SUTTON

Ulysses Press ⚱ Berkeley, CA
1998

This book has been written and published strictly for informational purposes, and in no way should it be used as a substitute for consultation with your medical doctor or other health care professional. All facts in this book came from medical files, clinical journals, scientific publications, personal interviews, published trade books, self-published materials by experts, magazine articles, and the personal-practice experiences of the authorities quoted or sources cited. You should not consider educational material herein to be the practice of medicine or to replace consultation with a physician or other medical practitioner. The author and publisher are providing you with information in this work so that you can have the knowledge and can choose, at your own risk, to act on that knowledge. The author and publisher also urge all readers to be aware of their health status and to consult health professionals before beginning any health program, including changes in dietary habits.

Published by: Ulysses Press
          P.O. Box 3440
          Berkeley, CA 94703-3440

Library of Congress Catalog Card Number: 97-61008

ISBN: 1-56975-082-3

Printed in Canada by Best Book Manufacturers

First published as *Healing with Shiatsu*, Gill & Macmillan, 1996

10 9 8 7 6 5 4 3 2 1

Editorial: Lily Chou
Typesetter: David Wells
Cover Design: B & L Design
Indexer: Sayre Van Young

Distributed in the United States by Publishers Group West and in Canada by Raincoast Books

TABLE OF CONTENTS

WHAT IS SHIATSU?

Shiatsu is one of many practices that help us to transform our lives through cultivating an awareness of ourselves and what brings about our negative states — and also what is required to create a more positive state. Its roots are in ancient Chinese massage, which employs theories and techniques from Chinese culture and philosophy to create wholeness and well-being. The Japanese word *shiatsu* means finger pressure: *shi* — "finger," *atsu* — "pressure." In shiatsu, the fingers, thumbs, elbows, knees and hands are all used to stimulate or sedate the energy flowing through the body to promote health and healing.

Shiatsu encourages a positive state of mind; its theories and techniques are a backdrop to physical communication through touch. Like acupuncture and other Asian medical practices, shiatsu works with the body's energy system. The Asian concept of energy can be loosely understood as "vitality" or "vital force," which we cannot see but can sense or feel. For example, if someone walks into the room we immediately pick up on his energetic state, whether he looks full of life and energy or the opposite. In this book, I will use "energy" and *ki* to describe this vital force.

According to Asian medicine, our energy, or *ki*, moves along specific pathways (meridians) around the body. These meridians relate to our internal physical organs and our emotional, psychological and spiritual state. The organs and functions in the body are divided into six pairs and all are linked by *ki*. For the Chinese, all parts and functions of the body are interrelated; no problem can successfully be treated in isolation. In shiatsu, the connecting point of the organs and functions in the body is the meridian system.

The Meridians

The meridians are like a closed circuit of water channels, and the water flowing through the channels is equivalent to the *ki*. There can be many interruptions along the way — sticks, stones and leaves silt up the channels, with a resulting blockage. If this keeps happening, the water will continue to be disrupted and blocked. On one side of the blockage there is too much water and on the other too little. The difference becomes more apparent the longer the blockages remain. Similarly, if we continue to deny the causes of our blockages our energy will decline. Our blockages can be felt as stagnation in the body, with the "full" side as a pain or discomfort and the "empty" side as a weakness or apathy. Inefficient flow of *ki* around the body results in tiredness, physical pain, depression, emotional upsets, stiffness, headaches and many more common problems. Various shiatsu techniques are used to correct these imbalances (see Chapter Seven).

Along the meridians are *tsubos*, or specific energy points, where the *ki* is more active; it is in here that blockages can be felt most clearly and where the energy can also be released. The *tsubos* are the same as Chinese acupuncture points. There are approximately 365 in total, although far fewer are used in shiatsu practice.

Shiatsu has a diagnostic element and can be used as a treatment or in the prevention of disease. The practice of shiatsu can still be very powerful, even without any true understanding of Chinese philosophy, the meridians or the energy system.

TRUST AND TOUCH

Much of the healing takes place through compassionate touch and listening, as well as the person allowing himself the time for treatment such as shiatsu. We can see this in the way a child wants a hug when she is in pain or feeling insecure — that magic kiss on a sore knee is better than any painkiller. As adults we experience comfort through touch, particularly when in difficulty. This touching is not learned behavior, but rather something instinctive.

A large part of the effectiveness of shiatsu is the trust between the practitioner and the receiver. With trust the receiver can relax and, in this state of relaxation, the body no longer needs to "hold on." Once this happens the reason for the holding on can come to the surface. Shiatsu can therefore be useful in getting to the underlying causes of physical and emotional discomfort. The more we push against the way things are the more resistance is built up; the more support we get the more trust we build.

There are many examples in daily life of the body tensing up, with resulting physical discomfort. If you talk to the bank manager about an overdraft or witness an unhappy scene, your body will tell you that this is not your favorite pastime! Different people have different areas that tend to hold tension when they find themselves in an uncomfortable situation. If the tension is felt in the shoulders, for instance, it is only a symptom of the cause — although they may be in agony, the shoulders themselves are not the problem. Tensions can be stored in different areas in the body for years, building up. Eventually a chronic state develops, resulting in permanent discomfort and disease. The shiatsu practitioner seeks to discover these tensions and blockages; once the cause is acknowledged healing can begin.

HOW CAN SHIATSU BE PRACTICED?

Shiatsu can be practiced on two different levels. The first is a "do it yourself" form — on friends, family and neighbors. It can be learned at a beginner's class or from a book. Although this form of shiatsu does not employ elaborate techniques, it can still be very effective. It can be used for a variety of ailments — for example, headaches, stiffness, aches and pains, tiredness and tension-related disorders.

The second form is professional shiatsu, which is practiced by those who have undergone a professional training program and have a recognized qualification. After two to three years training the professional therapist should be competent to deal with a wide variety of conditions.

In Japan, shiatsu is used much of the time as a preventative measure rather than as a treatment to "cure" illness. In the West, it is still used mainly for people who have been unwell and cannot seem to improve through conventional therapy. Shiatsu is slowly becoming appreciated as a positive way to maintain good health and happiness. Frequently, those who have experienced its benefits for a specific ailment use it regularly to enhance their well-being.

THE PHYSICAL BENEFITS OF SHIATSU

Shiatsu helps to maintain overall health and encourages people to listen more keenly to what the body is saying. With this increased awareness, it becomes easier to see what is wholesome and what is destructive, giving us choices about which path to follow. The body has a great ability to self-heal, but sometimes it needs assistance to remove the objects getting in the way of the healing process. Shiatsu is one technique that can help to remove these blockages.

WHAT CONDITIONS CAN SHIATSU HELP?

Because shiatsu works on the energetic system, it can be useful in helping a wide range of disorders. Bear in mind that not recognizing the laws of nature and living in an inharmonious way is contrary to what shiatsu promotes. A shiatsu treatment will be of maximum value if it is supported by an understanding of the cause of the condition, and if the person follows a moderate outlook and lifestyle.

Shiatsu can specifically help the following:

- arthritic conditions

- backaches

- emotional difficulties

- headaches/migraines

- insomnia

- intestinal disorders (irritable bowel syndrome, colitis, constipation and diarrhea)

- menstrual problems (heavy periods and premenstrual syndrome)

- muscular tensions

- reproductive problems (including endometriosis and fibroids)

- respiratory difficulties (asthma, bronchitis and recurrent chest infections)

- sinusitis

- stress-related disorders

Shiatsu is a catalyst in the healing process. Healing is not something that just sometimes "happens" — it is a continuous movement toward harmony, balance and wholeness.

WHAT HAPPENS DURING A SHIATSU MASSAGE?

When shiatsu is given, the skin surface is immediately stimulated, triggering a response in the nervous system. Any sensory stimulation is automatically picked up by the nervous system and then taken to the brain for interpretation.

The autonomic nervous system is the subconscious part of the nervous system and coordinates all involuntary movements and functions of the body. It is divided into two parts: the sympathetic and the parasympathetic nervous systems. Our way of being and feeling changes considerably depending on the relative balance of these two systems. Many influences — both internal and external — can tip this balance and cause dominance in one or other of the parts of the autonomic nervous system, resulting in a feeling of being out of sorts. The sympathetic branch of the nervous system is concerned with the stress response and preparation for fight or flight — when something stressful comes our way, the body tries to defend itself by either fighting or running away.

The changes that take place when the sympathetic nervous system is dominant are:

- the muscles contract to prepare for escape
- there is a feeling of alertness
- the pupils dilate
- the blood vessels contract
- the digestive system temporarily contracts
- the heartbeat increases
- the secretions in the mouth dry up
- the hair on the skin stands up
- the liver releases more glucose into the muscles

All these responses prepare the body for action. Once the immediate danger has gone, the parasympathetic nerves become the more dominant. All the systems start to return to normal and there is a feeling of relief, letting go and relaxation. The parasympathetic response is sometimes known as the peacemaker. There is a very fine point of balance between the two systems. We are constantly trying to maintain this balance, both consciously and subconsciously.

Much of the stress that we encounter today is not from an immediate and identifiable source — it is in the background, constantly niggling away. With this persistent, low-lying stress, the body is on the alert a lot of the time. As a result, the systems are always on the defensive, and a feeling of total relaxation is difficult to experience. Through shiatsu, we can encourage the body and mind to relax and let go of tension — to switch from sympathetic to parasympathetic dominance. Then it is possible to feel at peace, with clarity the oneness that is blocked so much of the time. This "being in the present moment" is the most restful place to abide. Using quiet and gentle movements, we can encourage the parasympathetic response; through more active, vigorous movements we can stimulate the sympathetic nervous system.

We can through shiatsu become aware of what happens with pain and soreness in the body. If pain is experienced, the immediate reaction is to tense up against it. This tightens the body, adding to the discomfort; it blocks the energy paths to the area so that valuable energy is not getting through to where it is needed. Shiatsu techniques help to relax muscle tightness, enabling the vital energy flow to be restored.

WHAT TO EXPECT IN A SHIATSU SESSION

A shiatsu session is a dynamic interchange of energy on many different levels. There is no rigid formula, but at first it is useful to have a framework within which to work. This framework gives confidence to the practitioner and a flow to the treatment. For the more experienced practitioner, the approach and style very much depend on his or her training, personality and area of interest. The aim is the same: to create balance physically, mentally and spiritually, and to allow the client space to open up and see the true cause for his or her present condition. This will take varying amounts of time, depending on the condition.

Shiatsu is done through the clothes, and a treatment — usually taking a little over an hour — is normally given on a thick mat on the floor. One session is not as beneficial as three or four spaced out over a period of four to six weeks. The number of sessions needed for any one individual depends on his or her particular problem. If the energy is very deficient, a number of sessions is desirable in order to monitor the changes taking place and to ensure that any advice given is of help.

CASE HISTORY

A session normally starts with the taking of a case history in order to get a picture of the present complaint in the context of the person's life. Questions are asked about the present complaint, past medical history, lifestyle, food habits, exercise, relaxation and anything else that may be significant.

DIAGNOSIS

Diagnosis of the problem is assisted in the following ways:

VISUAL DIAGNOSIS

This will include visual observations, posture, mannerisms, skin color and walk.

AUDITORY DIAGNOSIS

This will include seeing how the voice sounds — shaky, tense, timid, loud, etc.

TOUCH DIAGNOSIS

This is to access the quality of energy in the person.

The latter is normally done through a specific type of diagnosis called *hara* diagnosis (see Chapter Six). The *hara*, or abdomen, is palpated very gently to detect the areas of fullness and the areas that lack energy. A diagnosis can also be made by looking at different areas on the back, and by feeling the quality of energy in the meridians — again to detect areas of fullness or emptiness.

SHIATSU TECHNIQUES

When a diagnosis has been made a number of different techniques can be used to change the quality of the energy (see Chapter Seven). The techniques are basically stimulating or sedating.

The whole body can be worked on in shiatsu — with increased awareness and sensitivity the practitioner is drawn to the areas that need most attention. In obviously tense areas the *ki* is dispersed; in areas lacking in *ki* stimulating and holding techniques are used to encourage the flow of energy back to that area.

Often a weak area needs to be held for two or three minutes before the energy starts to fill it. It may appear that nothing is happening, but on a subtle level changes are taking place. Sometimes it is possible to feel such changes immediately and other times it is not until later that more energy is felt. The easiest area to feel and hear changes is in the abdomen when it starts to relax — a gurgling noise may be heard and a lot of movement is felt, which is the parasympathetic nervous system taking the dominant role.

A combination of techniques including stretching, pressing, holding and rotating are used to work on different areas of the body. Sometimes tense areas are present as a protection against an underlying emotional weakness; when the tension is dissolved the emotion may come to the surface, to a conscious level, often with an outburst followed by a sense of relief, tiredness, shivering or crying. When responded to compassionately, these feelings subside and a sense of well-being and peace takes over. The receiver will always feel better if the treatment is given with a loving, gentle attitude, and a genuine wish for this person to be well.

The primary encouragement to anyone receiving shiatsu is to try to live in a more harmonious way, with a mindfulness of daily actions and relationships. With a strengthened awareness we are more in control of what we do and say, and have a greater chance of performing positive actions rather than ones that harm ourselves, others and the world around us.

CONCLUDING THE SESSION

Usually at the end of a session the client will feel relaxed and energized, with a sense of calm, or sometimes wanting a long sleep. Normally there is a noticeable increase in flexibility and a decrease in muscular aches and pains. If the shiatsu treatment has triggered some emotional discomfort there may be feelings of sadness, anger or fear and the receiver may feel chilled (a blanket and a hot drink can help). The cooling down is due to letting go of tensions held in the muscles. There can be a feeling of lethargy because of deep work and release of energy, feelings and emotions. If those things that have been blocking the healing process are removed then over the next days and weeks changes will start to take place both on a conscious and subconscious level, with a resulting feeling of vibrance and freedom.

In order for the healing to continue, the practitioner may give advice on diet, lifestyle, environment or attitude (see Chapter Eight).

On leaving the treatment room the receiver should keep warm, and if possible rest for a short time.

2

THE HISTORY
OF SHIATSU

—

The term shiatsu came about in the twentieth century when there began to be a revival of some ancient healing practices. Yet when the nature of shiatsu is considered — finger pressure and body contact to relieve pain and discomfort — it will be appreciated that this instinctive approach to healing is as old as time, and far older than written records.

ANCIENT CHINA

The practice of rubbing, massaging and pressing the body to enhance well-being has its origins in ancient China. Massage was recognized for many years there as one of four forms of medical treatment, together with acupuncture, herbalism and moxabustion (using heat on specific areas to draw energy into them). Tradition relates that *anmo* — the practice of touching specific points on the body to encourage well-being — was first set down in the time of the Yellow Emperor (2697–2596 B.C.) in a text called the *Nei Ching* (often called *The Yellow Emperor's Classic of Internal Medicine*). In this book it is stated that "certain diseases and discomforts are best treated with massage and breathing exercises." Shiatsu has its roots in ancient Asian theory, which cannot be separated from Chinese philosophy (see Chapter Four).

THE ART OF ANMA

In the sixth century A.D., Buddhism was introduced into Japan, and with it came Chinese philosophy and culture. The art of anmo (known as *anma* in Japan) was introduced, along with other healing practices. One of these was tao-yinn, which is a series of exercises to improve health and sensory control. The combination of tao-yinn, massage and rubbing techniques was similar to what is known today as shiatsu.

In the 4500 years since some of these massage practices were recorded many changes have taken place. Despite this, however, the art of shiatsu has preserved its roots.

During the seventeenth century in Japan, it was declared that anma was to be practiced only by blind people since they had a very highly developed sense of touch. Because the blind were not well educated, anma was then practiced as an intuitive art, with little or no emphasis on technical and medical information. Doctors were required to practice anma for a time, though, in order to become familiar with human anatomy; to develop a feel for the energy in the body; and to locate the energy channel so that they could diagnose and treat with greater accuracy.

In the nineteenth century, anma developed into a therapy that treated muscular tensions and simple aches and pains; by the early twentieth century it had become licensed solely to promote pleasure and relaxation. Around this time, there were still people who wished to practice it as a "medical" way of treating illness. In order to separate themselves from the blind practitioners of anma they coined the term shiatsu. Practitioners of shiatsu were not subject to the restricted regulations that bound those giving anma.

SHIATSU IN THE TWENTIETH CENTURY

A man called Tamai Tempaka then wrote a book called *Shiatsu-Ho*. He brought together anma, *do-in* (self-shiatsu/massage), his studies in Western anatomy and physiology, massage and some of his own spiritual understandings. Three of his students were to become some of the best known shiatsu teachers of the twentieth century — Shizuto Masunaga, Tokujiro Namikoshi and Katsusuke Serizawa.

In the 1950s, shiatsu became officially recognized by the Japanese government. This came about because of a man called Namakoshi who in 1925 established a shiatsu training school. In his endeavor to get the practice officially accepted, he seems to have removed all references to the meridians from his teaching; much of the ancient traditional philosophy has been diluted and replaced with an emphasis on Western anatomy and the reflex points on the body.

Shizutzo Masunaga re-introduced a more traditional, philosophical and psychological framework into shiatsu practice. His main concern was to integrate Western philosophy and psychology with ancient Chinese tradition. Masunaga's interest in the energy channels for diagnosis and treatment revived the older art of ancient Chinese massage as a medical treatment.

SCHOOLS OF SHIATSU

Various schools and styles of shiatsu have arisen over the last forty years, the most notable of which are outlined below.

ZEN SHIATSU

This is based on Masunaga's style; it has less emphasis on *tsubos* and more on the meridian system, and the connection and change that is felt through the holding of two hands on the body. Masunaga introduced the concept of *kyo* and *jitsu* to assess the quality of energy in the body. Zen shiatsu not only works with the twelve classical meridians familiar to shiatsu and acupuncture, but also uses the "extended" meridian system, which includes an additional twelve meridians.

OHASHIATSU

This style of shiatsu is based on the teaching of Wataru Ohashi. It relies on using the twelve traditional energy channels and *tsubos* to change the energy in the body. It also incorporates some of Masunaga's shiatsu and much of Ohashi's own individual style.

NIPPON

The teachings of Namakoshi form the basis of this style of shiatsu. There is great emphasis on Western anatomy and physiology and reflex points.

MACROBIOTIC SHIATSU

This incorporates the twelve classical meridians and a way of living in harmony with the world as taught originally by George Ohsawa.

FIVE ELEMENTS SHIATSU

This is based on the five elements theory as understood in traditional Chinese medicine.

There are hundreds of shiatsu schools around the world, most of which have opened in the 1980s and 1990s. Each school has its own value, unique style and emphasis.

Over the years I have developed my own way of working with shiatsu, incorporating a strong influence from the training I had in Zen shiatsu and Ohashiatsu together with my own commitment to exploring a spiritual path.

3

SICKNESS AND THE
HEALING PROCESS

———

Disharmony in the body and mind that creates discomfort and pain is what we call illness. Illness can be seen as part of a natural process. Along with old age and death, it is guaranteed to most of us. We will all die, so does it follow that we will frequently experience sickness, too? It seems that way. Yet many stress-related diseases, those resulting from substance abuse, poor nutrition, an unhealthy environment, unwholesome states of mind and infectious diseases, all contribute to people dying young. Some can surely be prevented.

We spend little time reflecting on the extraordinary way that our bodies and minds work — we take them for granted. We do, however, spend a lot of time thinking about how we would like them to be — less painful, fitter, taller, healthier, fatter, thinner, less confused, more intelligent. This lack of true awareness leads to inappropriate habits that contribute to ill health. Good health is a little like happiness — we tend not to notice we have it until it is gone. When we lose it, we realize how precious it was.

WHAT CREATES DISHARMONY IN THE BODY/MIND?

GREED OR OVERINDULGENCE

Overindulgence is often thought of in the context of food, but it includes excesses on the physical, mental and emotional levels as well. Greed is about wanting things we don't have, and about not wanting to let go of things that we do have. This creates a tight grip, a tension that can block many functions in the body. The tension then manifests in discomfort and disease — a headache or stomach ache being two obvious examples. Too much food contributes to health problems such as obesity, diabetes and heart disease; too much external pollution, cigarette smoking, alcohol and drugs create other problems. Very strong emotions also lead to destruction of the body and mind.

DISSATISFACTION

Not being content with the way things are can set up a continuous struggle and create inner tension. Under these circumstances we cannot rest and enjoy a peaceful life; instead, the resulting tension leads to discomfort and disease.

DELUSION

For a human being who has not yet reached enlightenment, delusion is easy to suffer from! We spend little time considering the natural order of things, developing wisdom and the ability to see reality clearly.

INHERITED TENDENCIES

It is often difficult to accept illness, particularly in children. There are no definitive explanations, but we are born with inherited tendencies of which we should become more aware. An understanding of rebirth and the law of karma (that every action and attitude has a cause and effect) can help us to accept these predispositions more easily.

Some people are born with a strong constitution and others seem to be sickly from an early age. Those with a weak make up have to make a greater effort to stay well, while the stronger can get away with more abuse — but not forever! Our inherited constitution is one thing, but our present condition is quite another. How we live and think creates the latter condition; we have more control over it than our genes (see Chapter Four). Our condition results from how we nourish ourselves — physically, mentally and spiritually. By developing more awareness and by living mindfully, we can live more harmoniously with ourselves and others.

WHY SHIATSU?

I chose to study shiatsu because it seemed to me a reasonably "whole" way of looking at health. I trained as a nurse and midwife, but nursing never took the opportunity to properly examine sickness and how the individual is involved in the process (and to a degree responsible for it).

I was then fortunate enough to spend twenty-seven months in a very remote part of Papua New Guinea running a small bush hospital. While there, I started to see the relationship between body and mind, and that we do have some choice about how well or sick we are. I witnessed the power that the mind has over the body through traditional healing practices and bush medicine. I saw people developing sore throats because they had stolen food from someone's garden — the sore throat being a "punishment." I saw others develop high fevers from "spells" that had been cast over them for a wrongdoing. People truly believed that they had had inner organs removed and replaced with wood or some other natural elements in bush operations.

During my stay, I was extremely healthy and had plenty of energy while eating a simple diet accompanied by a lot of exercise. Back in Ireland I noticed the stark contrast of overindulging in so many things and the resulting problems. I then wanted to study a healing practice that would allow me to truly connect with people, and to try and understand illness and our role in it. Through shiatsu I found the opportunity to view a person as a whole — body, mind, emotions and spirit. I saw touch as a powerful way to help a person learn to listen to his or her own body and find a natural rhythm.

While I appreciate the Chinese culture from which shiatsu has arisen, and the philosophy and lifestyle that supports it, I sometimes find it difficult to believe wholeheartedly that shiatsu works as it does. The concept that energy running up and down the meridians is so easily influenced merely by touch seems too simple — but it certainly appears to work. However, many factors are important in the process of healing and these need to be considered as well as the practical techniques of shiatsu.

WHAT IS HEALING?

In *Relaxation, Concentration and Meditation* by Joel Levey, George Leonard is quoted: "At the heart of each of us, whatever our imperfections, there exists a silent pulse of perfect rhythm — a complex of wave forms and resonances which is absolutely individual and unique and yet which connects us to everything in the universe." To heal means to become whole. If you consider this, healing is about becoming complete, total, at one or unified. It is quite an ambitious task! It may be more realistic to see healing as a process that leads us through life.

The word for health in Chinese is composed of two characters. The first describes a human being standing upright and the second describes someone at ease and relaxed after all extraneous things have been dispensed with. This is another way of saying that health means finding balance in life by giving up or letting go of unnecessary baggage.

As an evolutionary necessity animals have had to have some kind of healing system to counteract the forces that attack both internally and externally to create illness, injury and shock. The very survival of a species implies a healing system. The body has a built-in power that heals and restores balance, but it can only cope with a certain amount of abuse before it starts to give out signals to make some changes. No drugs or intervention can encourage healing if the body is not in a position to respond. The basic make up of the body has not changed for many thousands of years, yet what it is subjected to in the way of unnatural foods, environmental factors and stress is increasing daily. With these adverse changes the healing system comes under threat.

How Does Healing Occur?

Healing takes place on a number of levels, the first being on the physical plane through the immune system and the action of white blood cells and antibodies. A strong and efficient immune system is dependent on many factors — good nutrition, a low stress level, a positive attitude toward life, and a clean environment.

The second level is more subtle and concerns the mind. It involves faith in a power that can heal, coming either from within or outside, and an acceptance of where we are right now. Faith in the healing power of a person (self or other) and faith in an object can be responsible for healing. This is the function of placebos, sacred shrines, faith healers and positive mind states. Healing *does* take place when placebos are given and when people pray at shrines, go to faith healers or develop very positive mental attitudes. The trust and belief that healing is possible allows the individual to let go of pain, sickness or emotional trauma.

With a more relaxed attitude the system is not under such stress, and a natural healing response can start to take place. There is no longer the need to take a defensive stance toward life. When a person is in a relaxed frame of mind the natural rhythm of the body can more easily be restored. Most people do not go through life in an "accepting mode." Instead, they are often confrontational, trying to change the way things are and to control situations thereby creating an enormous amount of pressure. This way of living is not conducive to a natural healing response. The energy required to hold down emotions or to deal with excesses could be better used to heal ourselves. Acceptance can be the master key that unlocks healing, and the mind has an important role to play in this process.

So why do we get sick if we have a system that naturally regenerates and creates balance? The capacity of the healing system to keep and restore the balance of health is often exceeded by either external or internal forces, physical or emotional. The body and mind are constantly being filled with things that are in excess of their basic requirements, and the ability to process and cope with these excesses is constantly being challenged. We develop habitual ways of reacting, which get stronger as we reinforce them over time. If they are creating negativity, this is ingrained in our being, creating destruction and disharmony.

As I mentioned above, excesses are not only on a physical level but on an emotional level as well. Too many uncontrolled feelings, strong attachments to ideas and possessions cause destruction in the body. If we can remove the obstacles that are preventing healing, the healing process and immune system can do the work. But first the excesses have to be observed, and then some intelligent choices made about how to live in a more balanced way. It can be a challenge to use sickness as a opportunity to transform. To try and accept the illness and relax with it enhances the power of healing.

CAN ILLNESS BE POSITIVE?

If you feel unwell, ask yourself the following questions:

- What can I learn from this illness?

- Why am I sick?

- What can I do to be well?

- What am I holding on to that is creating tension and discomfort?

By reflecting in this way we can see a more positive side to illness. This can be encouraged and supported through regular shiatsu sessions where the practitioner can make observations and recommend guidelines for change. Ajhan Chah writes:

- Do everything with a mind that lets go.

- Do not expect any praise or reward.

- If you let go a little, you will have a little peace.

- If you let go a lot, you will have a lot of peace.

- If you let go completely, you will know complete peace and freedom.

- Your struggles with the world will have come to an end.

4

EASTERN PHILOSOPHY

Eastern philosophy, with its roots in China, is vast and complex. In this book, I will touch on some of its aspects in order to put the roots of shiatsu in context. The ideas fundamental to Eastern philosophy, and useful in understanding shiatsu, are:

- the concept of *ki* energy
- the concept of yin and yang
- the concept of the tao
- the theory of the five elements, five phases or five transformations.

KI

The word *ki* (*qi* in Chinese) is very commonly used in China and Japan. It refers to that which binds, forms, animates and unifies energy into matter — *ki* is a cohesive force and without it there would be no tangible matter, no form, no concrete substances. Everything in the universe, both organic and inorganic, is defined by its *ki*.

The life essence within matter is known as *jing* or "essence." The difference between the living and the non-living is the presence of *jing*; it enables the process of birth, life and death. *Jing* is stored in the kidneys and accounts for our constitutional strength (which we are born with). *Jing* is the source of life. *Ki* is the ability to activate and move.

Shen is the energy behind human consciousness; it enables us to think and discriminate and it determines personality. It is the vitality behind both *jing* and *ki* in the human body.

In shiatsu, we try to balance the *ki* energy to bring the body/mind back to a state of harmony. *Ki* can be seen in very subtle forms like emotions and feelings, or in grosser forms like trees, storms, rocks, oceans and the human body. *Ki*, which permeates everything, is in a constant state of change. In a busy day we tend not to be in touch with the natural forces around us, and do not see the interplay of forces keeping a natural rhythm in the universe or in ourselves as individuals. The constant ebb and flow of *ki* keeps us, and everything around us, alive.

Ki is not just the "vital energy" it is often translated as. Chinese philosophy does not speculate (as we do) about what *ki* is — it sees this force for what it does. Traditionally, the force of *ki* can be seen in three ways:

- prenatal *ki* — our inherited *ki* or energy
- grain *ki* — energy taken in from food
- natural air *ki* — energy taken in from the air

The combination of all three is normal *ki*.

THE PURPOSE OF NORMAL KI

How well we use *ki* depends on how we live our lives and on our attitudes. The more we live in harmony with natural forces and the more aware we are of our every action, the more harmonious our *ki* will be. Normal *ki* has five basic functions within the body:

- movement — general activity
- protection — protects from outside influences
- retention — holding on to substances for use; the holding of organs in place
- transformation — what we take in through food and air is transformed
- warms — keeps heat in the body

In shiatsu, we try to access the state of *ki* in a person through various methods of diagnosis, and then use techniques to rebalance it as necessary.

YIN AND YANG

Yin and yang represent complementary polar opposites that are constantly shifting and changing; they are also interdependent. They can be observed in almost anything we look at — day changing into night, winter into spring, youth into old age, hot into cold, happiness into sadness. This understanding of the interchanging of everything permeates the social, medical and philosophical cultures of the East.

Although we live in a world of opposites, in the West we see opposites as divorced from one another rather than as two parts of a whole. We have a tendency to compartmentalize things. For example, buying and selling are two opposites of one event yet we usually see them as totally different. If you buy something, though, someone else is selling it. In the same way, all opposites share an implicit identity.

We tend to create boundaries around things rather than seeing everything as a part of a greater whole. We say "this is the shore" and "this is the sea"; immediately we have a division. Rather than seeing that the line where the sea touches the shore is where they unite and join we see it as where it divides and separates. Everything is in a constant state of flux; even the densest piece of rock is slowly changing into sand and the most solid mountain is gradually being eroded.

The Chinese characters for yin and yang originated from observing a hillside. Yin was the shady side of the hill and yang the sunny side. By looking at the qualities of these positions on a hillside, we can see some of the properties yin and yang represent.

YANG (SUNNY SIDE)	YIN (SHADY SIDE)
light	dark
outside	inside
heat	cold
heaven	earth
dry	wet
fire	water
sun	moon
expansion	contraction

These qualities relate not only to tangible phenomena outside the body, but also to internal and more subtle movements. Yin and yang can be applied to anything, and below you can see the theory applied to human personality and physiology.

YANG	YIN
warm body	cool body
warm personality	cool personality
dry skin	moist skin
outgoing	introverted
positive	negative
aggressive	timid
angry and impatient	fearful and insecure

speedy	lazy
desirous	complacent
tense and strong	flaccid and weak

YIN AND YANG AND SHIATSU

Yin and yang can be used as a general guide to access the state of a person's *ki*. In shiatsu, a diagnosis is made by assessing the energetic quality of the person rather than by relying on Western diagnostic techniques. If a person is too active, he or she needs more of the opposite, more rest; if too angry, more compassion is needed; if too fearful, more attention and security.

We strive to find the middle way of balance or harmony. We can do this through our natural instincts, but also through more careful observation and attention to ourselves. Yin and yang are descriptive techniques that can help to alert us to the way in which we are living our lives. With better observation, we can then endeavor to return to the tao — the natural way.

TAO

Tao is loosely translated as "the way" — there is no precise Western term for it. It is the interplay of forces in the universe; by living in harmony with these forces we can live in harmony with nature. According to the tao, we can achieve higher states of being — otherwise we become out of harmony, dissatisfied and ill. Taoism has been a part of Asian culture for thousands of years, but it became more formalized around the sixth century B.C. Lao Tzu's *Tao Te Ching* is one of its main texts.

THE THEORY OF THE FIVE ELEMENTS

This way of categorizing phenomena was a later addition to the theory of yin and yang, and was not documented until around the fourth century B.C. It is a complex theory that was probably in gestation for many years before finally being written down. It is an explanatory theory, not a doctrine. It can be useful as a guide to clinical tendencies and to see patterns in a person, but the ultimate test is in the *overall* pattern that is observed.

The five elements theory reflects the rhythms of nature and can be seen to affect a wide range of things — agriculture, nutrition, psychology, philosophy and the human body. Each element can be related to a different organ and function in the body — a season, a time of year, a feeling, a taste and a sound, to name but a few of the associations. In this way of looking at the world, the five elements of wood, fire, earth, metal and water are seen as categories into which all things and events in the universe can be organized. These categories were never intended to be taken literally, but instead used to describe the changing patterns; functions and qualities of phenomena in the world.

CREATIVE AND DESTRUCTIVE CYCLES

A continuous cycle can be observed, with the energy changing from one element to the next. The most active part of the cycle is the energy of fire, represented in the body by the heart and small intestine. The fire is hot and active like the summer sun, but it eventually burns down to form ashes. As it starts to contract and cool, it creates the next phase, soil or earth. The ashes of the fire decompose into soil — this phase is represented by the stomach and spleen.

The energy continues to contract and change, with the extreme contraction leading to the next phase — metal. Metal is a very strong substance found deep in the ground. The metal phase is represented in the body by the lungs and large intestine. When this solidification reaches an extreme, it starts to expand again and eventually liquifies and leads to the water phase of the cycle, represented by the kidneys and bladder. This phase is like winter — cool, with a lot of moisture. The water starts to disperse outward and flow to nourish plants and trees. Things then start the growth common to spring time, and this tree or wood energy is represented in the body by the liver and gall bladder. The movement at this phase is very active again, moving upward and outward. The energy then reaches its peak, and the cycle starts again with fire.

This cycle is known as the *shen*, or creative/supportive cycle. At each stage there is a particular energy which in turn transforms into the next phase of the cycle, having been created by the previous phase. There is also a control or destructive cycle, known as the *ko* cycle (see Illustration 1). In this cycle, we can see how overactivity in one phase can result in imbalance in another phase:

- overstimulation or disharmony of the rising wood element affects the gathering soil energy
- overstimulation of the gathering soil energy interferes with the relaxing quality of the water
- overstimulation of the water energy slows down the fire
- overstimulation of fire prevents consolidation of the metal part of the cycle
- consolidating metal energy affects the rising of tree energy.

The supportive or creative cycle can be seen by thinking of how:

- *wood* burns to make
- *fire*, whose ashes decompose into the
- *earth* where are born and mined
- *metals* which when melted become
- *water* which nourishes trees and plants.

The control or destructive cycle can be seen in the following:

- *wood* is cut down by *metal*
- *fire* is extinguished by *water*

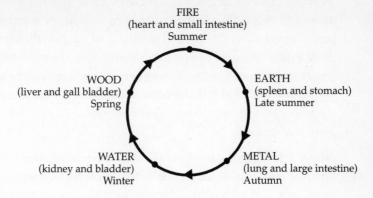

Creative or Shen Cycle

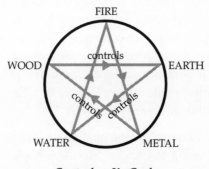

Control or Ko Cycle

Illustration 1: Creative or Shen Cycle & Control or Ko Cycle

- *earth* is penetrated by *wood*
- *metal* is melted by *fire*
- *water* is interrupted and cut off by *earth*.

OTHER ASPECTS OF EXISTENCE

Another application of the five elements theory is found in relation to the seasons. Wood is seen as the spring, when everything starts to grow and there is a real upward movement of energy. Fire is the summer, with a lot of heat and activity and everything is at the height of its growth. Metal is like autumn, when everything starts to contract and get ready for a quiet winter — the energy is one of turning inward and downward. Water represents winter, a time for rest and decisions about change. Earth represents the transition between seasons.

Many other aspects of existence have been associated with the five elements — for example, the emotions of anger, joy, grief, fear and sympathy, which in turn are associated with wood, fire, metal, water and earth. The same goes for tastes, skin color and sounds.

All these ideas permeate Chinese thought, culture, medicine and philosophy. If understood correctly, they can make shiatsu very exciting. Through the five elements, we can see the endless unfolding of energy and constantly changing nature of things. After some time working with the five elements, it becomes easier to see patterns in people and to make appropriate suggestions as to what may best help to change the imbalances observed.

You can elaborate on the qualities that each element expresses by looking at Chapter Five, The Meridians; each pair of meridians is associated with one of the five elements. Through studying and observing how different qualities and characteristics fit into the five-element cycle, it is then possible to use the cycle as a way of diagnosing conditions and seeing which associated elements can have a positive or negative effect and thus influence healing (see Chapter Six, Diagnosis).

Like any theory that categorizes people and things into different types, there is a tendency to pigeonhole! The intention of shiatsu and other Asian therapies is to observe very closely the everchanging nature of things and the impermanence of our human existence.

5

THE MERIDIANS

Our understanding of the meridians has developed over centuries of observation and practice. The word meridian means "a thread in a fabric" and "something that connects." The meridians are channels or pathways through which *ki* flows, giving nourishment and strength throughout the body. Each meridian is closely associated with a major organ or bodily function.

The energy from each of the organs is associated with a meridian; the energy from each meridian in turn connects with another, making a complete circuit. If all the channels are kept open and free of blockages, there will be no stagnation — there will instead be a feeling of vibrance on all levels.

Shiatsu aims to encourage a free flow of energy through these pathways. This can be done most satisfactorily with some input and effort on the part of the client.

The meridians can be felt in different ways, through developing both sensitivity and patience. They are not physical structures that continue on after death and then decay. Once life has left the body, the meridians cease to have a function.

The meridians also have an association with emotional and psychological conditions. Various imbalances in the organs not only affect us physically but also emotionally and psychologically. The same is true in the reverse. If we have an emotional or psychological upset, the physical body will also react. Over the years, emotional and psychological patterns have become associated with different organs and meridians.

Along the meridians there are *tsubos*, pressure or acupuncture points, where the energy is more active. Since we are dealing with a circuit of energy, if one meridian is out of harmony or balance, inevitably there will be a cumulative effect. If there is a lack of *ki* in one area there will be a fullness somewhere else. In shiatsu, we call this emptiness a *kyo* area, and the fullness is described as being *jitsu* (see Chapter Six).

THE SIX PAIRS OF MERIDIANS

In the most straightforward approach to shiatsu, there are twelve meridians, organized into six pairs:

- lungs and large intestine
- stomach and spleen
- heart and small intestine
- bladder and kidney
- heart governor and triple heater
- gall bladder and liver.

The pairs have complementary functions — one a yin function and its opposite a yang function (see Chapter Four). Two meridians are not really associated with an organ, but can be described as being connected with a system in the body. The first is the heart constrictor, heart governor or heart protector meridian. It is associated with the covering of the heart, the pericardium. Its main function is to protect the heart against external invasion and to govern the blood or circulatory system.

The second is the triple heater or triple warmer. This does not have a precise physical form or an association with any physical organ or structure. It is associated with "three burners," which equate to three chakras — the heart, the solar plexus and the *tanden* (the tanden is the energetic center of the body below the navel). The triple heater is responsible for producing and regulating the heat in the body. Two other channels — the governing vessel and the conception vessel — oversee the flow of energy in the meridians. The governing vessel influences all the yang meridians and the conception vessel the yin meridians.

I have chosen to highlight some of the aspects of each meridian that are common and easy to identify with. You may notice that you can closely identify with a certain set of conditions or characteristics associated with a particular meridian. This may indicate that there is a weakness, or a strength, in this part of your make-up.

Each pair of meridians is associated with one of the five elements — earth, wood, fire, metal and water. You will see certain personality types in each meridian description; you can then fit these into the five-element cycle and see the person and condition in the context of the *ko* or *shen* cycle (see Chapter Four).

The order in which I have listed the meridians follows the circuit through which they flow.

LUNGS AND LARGE INTESTINE

Element: Metal

Main Functions: Exchange, elimination and ability to create boundaries.

LUNGS

Controls: Intake of oxygen and *ki*; elimination of carbon dioxide; intake of new facts and influences around us.

Physical Associations: Lungs; nose; skin.

Psychological Associations: Openness; awareness; ability to create space and boundaries for oneself.

Physical Imbalances: Poor respiration and resulting lung disorders; shortness of breath; lack of vitality and weak voice; poor skin and skin disorders such as eczema.

Psychological Imbalances: Melancholy; withdrawn feelings; isolation and depression.

LARGE INTESTINE

Controls: Elimination (absorbs water and excretes feces as the end process of digestion); ability to hold on or let go as appropriate.

Physical Associations: Large bowel; skin; sinuses.

Psychological Associations: Ability to let go and move on.

Physical Imbalances: Any bowel disorders, including diarrhea, constipation, irritable bowel syndrome; skin disorders; overproduction of mucus.

Psychological Imbalances: Holding on to things (emotional and physical), an inability to let go.

STOMACH AND SPLEEN

Element: Earth

Main Functions: Ingestion and digestion; thinking process.

STOMACH

Controls: Intake of food and other nourishment such as information — digesting and making sense of it.

Physical Associations: Upper digestive tract (stomach in particular); control of appetite; the breasts; ovaries; lactation.

Psychological Associations: Thinking process — ideas and intellect; ability to be in harmony with the earth and to feel well grounded.

Physical Imbalances: Difficulty in converting food into energy; ulcers; indigestion; nausea; anorexia; breast cysts and uterine problems.

Psychological Imbalances: Worry over small things, with tension building up in the shoulders; not feeling grounded; obsessions and anxiety.

SPLEEN

Controls: Transformation of food and drink into *ki* energy; transportation of nutrients to other parts of the body.

Physical Associations: Digestive enzymes; appetite; muscle strength; the menstrual cycle.

Psychological Associations: Ideas and opinions, the thinking process and concentration.

Physical Imbalances: Any of the common upper digestive problems; menstrual problems; weight problems and lack of appetite.

Psychological Imbalances: Too much thinking and mental confusion; inability to digest information and usefully use it.

HEART AND SMALL INTESTINE

Element: Fire

Main Functions: Conversion and integration.

HEART

Controls: Circulation of blood; awareness (in Oriental medicine, the heart is said to house the mind).

Physical Associations: Heart; tongue; central nervous system; sweating.

Psychological Associations: Awareness; compassion; capacity for fun, joy, laughter; ability to communicate and think clearly.

Physical Imbalances: Heart and circulatory problems; palpitations; excessive sweating; speech problems.

Psychological Imbalances: Emotional instability; lack of compassion; hysteria; inability to communicate; memory problems; nervous excitement.

Small Intestine

Controls: Assimilation and absorption of nutrients; continues process of transforming food into ki.

Physical Associations: Small intestine; tongue; lower lip.

Psychological Associations: Determination; clarity in judgment and discrimination.

Physical Imbalances: Poor absorption of nutrients with resulting anemia and weakness.

Psychological Imbalances: Holding emotions such as anger and shock inside; inability to make decisions.

Bladder and Kidneys

Element: Water

Main Functions: Purification and regulation.

Bladder

Controls: Transformation, storage and excretion of fluids.

Physical Associations: Urinary system; bones; hair; teeth; autonomic nervous system; pituitary gland (which governs the endocrine system).

Psychological Associations: Courage; flexibility (of mind and body).

Physical Imbalances: Urinary tract problems; bone disease — osteoporosis; poor teeth; baldness; malfunction of autonomic nervous system, leading to either overreaction to stress or complacency.

Psychological Imbalances: Fear; timidity; restlessness.

KIDNEY

Controls: Manufacture of urine; maintenance of fluid balance in the body; stores the essence that governs the process of birth, development, and decay; autonomic nervous system; will power; sexual energy.

Physical Associations: The kidneys, ears, bones, teeth, the endocrine glands, sexual drive and inherited tendencies.

Psychological Associations: Courage, will power, ability to move forward.

Physical Imbalances: Kidney disorders; genetic defects; disorders of the endocrine system; some reproductive and sexual problems; fluid retention; weakness of the bones and teeth; hearing problems.

Psychological Imbalances: Fears and phobias; lack of will power and determination.

HEART CONSTRICTOR AND TRIPLE HEATER

Main Functions: Circulation and protection.

HEART CONSTRICTOR

Controls: Circulatory system; protects the heart.

Physical Associations: Heart and blood vessels.

Psychological Associations: Protection of the mind and emotions; ability to relate to others.

Physical Imbalances: Circulatory disorders — angina, varicose veins and poor circulation.

Psychological Imbalances: Insomnia; excessive dreaming; emotional vulnerability; exhaustion from concentrating too hard and difficulty in relating to others.

TRIPLE HEATER

Controls: Heating of organs through distributing *ki* from the *hara*; lymphatic flow; regulates distribution of nutrients to extremities.

Physical Associations: Organs located in the chest, the mid-abdominal region and those in the lower abdominal cavity.

Psychological Associations: Ability to interact with people.

Physical imbalances: Feelings of cold; low resistance to infections; lymphatic disorders.

Psychological imbalances: Difficulty in social situations; inability to warm and to get close to people.

LIVER AND GALL BLADDER

Element: Wood

Main Functions: Storage, distribution and smooth flow of *ki*.

LIVER

Controls: Storage and release of nutrients for distribution; breakdown of toxic substances.

Physical Associations: Liver; ligaments; tendons; eyes; detoxification; sugar metabolism.

Psychological Associations: Control; anger; ability to plan.

Physical imbalances: Liver disease; excess of toxins in the blood; migraine headache; stiffness in joints and ligaments; eye problems.

Psychological imbalances: Anger; rage; over-controlled emotions; rigid thoughts; overplanning.

GALL BLADDER

Controls: Storage and distribution of bile; judgment.

Physical Associations: Gall bladder; break down of fats; eyes.

Psychological Associations: Practical application of ideas; decision-making; responsibility; irritability.

Physical imbalances: Poor digestion of fatty foods; biliousness; gallstones; physical inflexibility.

Psychological imbalances: Indecision; lack of imagination and creativity; frustration; bitterness; fear of making decisions.

GOVERNING VESSEL

Controls: Yang meridians; carries yang energy to the meridians.

Physical Associations: Spine; brain; brings yang energy to the meridians.

Physical Imbalances: Back problems; disorders of the central nervous system.

Psychological Associations: General emotional sensitivity.

Psychological Imbalances: Sexual problems; lack of *ki*; nervous disorders.

CONCEPTION VESSEL

Controls: Yin meridians; reproductive system.

Physical Associations: Fertility; female reproductive system; abdomen; lungs; carries yin energy to the meridians.

Physical Imbalances: Reproductive problems; general weakness.

Psychological Associations: General communication; how we relate spiritually.

Psychological Imbalances: Lack of will power; difficulty in communicating and in sexual relationships.

The governing and conception vessels together are referred to as the central or spiritual channel. All the yang meridians are connected internally to the spiritual channel along the governing vessel; all the yin meridians along the conception vessel. The twelve classical meridians receive energy from and give excess energy to these vessels according to the body's needs.

6

DIAGNOSIS

For the beginner, diagnosis can be a threatening prospect. This book is not designed to give you a great deal of information on diagnosis, but rather to encourage you to increase your normal powers of observation. If these are sharpened, it is often sufficient for the beginner to be able to give a basic shiatsu treatment and some simple guidelines to assist healing.

Diagnosis in shiatsu is based on sharp observation and an interpretation of this observation into a useful treatment. For example, if you find that someone is tense and hyperactive, it makes sense to do a lot of work that will encourage them to slow down and relax. On the other hand, if a client is very lethargic, it is more appropriate to use techniques to encourage the movement of *ki* around the body.

As I have mentioned earlier in the book, in shiatsu we diagnose the energetic quality of the person rather than the physical condition of the actual organs and structures.

FORMS OF DIAGNOSIS

VISUAL

This means observing skin color, posture, way of sitting, general disposition, and ability to communicate. In addition there is the immediate, intuitive feeling you may pick up.

HEARING

Observing the tone of voice, speed of speech, flow and content of words.

QUESTIONING

Asking relevant questions may give you more insight into the nature of the person. This will include questions on life history, present condition, lifestyle, likes and dislikes.

TOUCH

Using gentle, mindful touch to access the state of *ki* energy in the various meridians.

The two simplest and most useful tools for diagnosing the state of *ki* are *kyo* and *jitsu*, and back diagnosis (see below).

KYO AND JITSU

These terms are used to describe the quality and degree of the *ki* and its intensity in the body. *Kyo* is a description of deficient energy and a feeling of emptiness or dissatisfaction. It also suggests being hidden, or not immediately apparent. *Jitsu* describes excess, fullness and overactive energy. It is easily seen, as it stands out rather than being hidden like *kyo*. Observing *kyo* and *jitsu* is a useful way of assessing the state of the energy in the body and in this way it can be used as a tool for diagnosis and treatment.

Recognizing energy balances

Kyo and *jitsu* have different tendencies and neither is a fixed state in the body — the quality of both is constantly changing. Recognizing *kyo* and *jitsu* states enables us to interpret the language of energy and develop the ability to recognize either too much or too little energy. With these two basic observations it will become more apparent with time that there are many variations of "too much" and "too little."

This assessment of the energetic quality is made by touching, listening and looking. It is not difficult to recognize someone who is bubbling with energy and restless. It is also reasonably easy to work out when a person is very depressed and troubled, with low energy. Once you start to notice the more extreme qualities it becomes easier to identify the subtle tendencies in people. (These observations need not, of course, be confined to giving a shiatsu treatment.)

You cannot have a *kyo* without a *jitsu* — they exist hand-in-hand, although one is usually more apparent than the other. If there is a *kyo* condition of weakness, emptiness and wanting (either physically or emotionally), this usually creates a need for some other function in the body to become more active or full — *jitsu* — in order to compensate.

Once the most obvious energy imbalances have been identified, it is then necessary to try to correct them in order to create an overall balance in the body. Since a *kyo* area means there is a deficiency of energy, you need to increase the energy to this place; likewise, if there is too much energy somewhere you need to disperse it. There are various techniques employed to increase or decrease energy as required (see Chapter Eight).

Working on kyo and jitsu

Pain in a *jitsu* area is not as uncomfortable as that felt in a *kyo* area because it tends to be more superficial. It is usually because of a *kyo* that the *jitsu* occurs, so it is a result and not a cause. The cause gives more discomfort than its effect.

Generally speaking, it is better to work on the *kyo* area first. You are thereby energizing an area of little energy, and in so doing you will usually notice that the *jitsu* area is less remarkable when you have finished — some energy has dispersed to the *kyo* from the *jitsu*. A *kyo* area can be quite tender and sensitive so it has to be treated with care. The technique used to encourage a *kyo* to relax, open and fill up is gentle yet firm, supporting pressure. Very careful and slow stretches are also useful to tone such an area. If there is very little *ki* in the place you are working on, you may need to hold it for many minutes before you feel any change. Once more *ki* energy is received, there can be a feeling of relief, vibrance and relaxation in the body.

If you work on a *jitsu* area first, it may be that the *ki* energy will be focused more toward this part; you may end up taking *ki* from the already *kyo* area, which may therefore be further depleted. By toning a *kyo* area first, you are lessening the intensity in the *jitsu* part. By working on a *jitsu* area we want to scatter the energy away from it, which is done by vigorous stretches, pummeling, deep and quick movements, shaking and rubbing.

Changing the energy in a *kyo* area is known as tonification.

Changing the energy in a *jitsu* area is called sedation.

Tonification usually helps the whole body, whereas sedation techniques are normally more localized.

EXAMPLES OF KYO AND JITSU

KYO	JITSU
empty	full
hidden	projecting
sunken	raised

deep	superficial
weakness	resistance
underactive, leading	overactive, leading
to stiffness	to blockage
slow to respond	quick to respond

The Hara

In professional shiatsu, *kyo* and *jitsu* used as a way of diagnosis are best assessed in the *hara*, the area normally referred to as the abdomen. It is found below the ribs and above the pelvis and is not protected by bone. It is here that the *ki* energy is stored and it is the center of balance of the body (see *hara* shiatsu in Chapter Eight). Because most of the major organs are in this region or in close contact with it, it is a good place for us to assess the energetic quality of the internal functions. Illustration 2 is like a map of the *hara* —

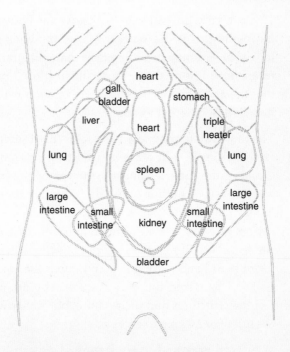

Illustration 2: Hara Diagnostic Areas

you can see the different diagnostic areas relating to the internal organs and functions. In these, the quality of the energy can be felt and then this information interpreted and used by the practitioner.

You can gently palpate the diagnostic areas of the *hara* by just touching the surface (not pressing) and working around it in a clockwise direction. As you do so, see if there is any noticeable difference from one area to the next, and if so make a mental note of it (but do not try to analyze it at this stage). This is known as a *hara* diagnosis. When this diagnosis has been done and other information obtained, the most *kyo* area is then worked on to improve the quality of energy there.

Once this has been done, the rest of the body will begin to feel more relaxed, balanced and tonified.

BACK DIAGNOSIS

This is a very general way to observe the body and what is happening in it. As with the *hara*, the back can also be looked at as a map recording facts that will guide us to some interesting information. From Illustration 3, you will see that the areas for diagnosis are the same in name as for the hara, but in different locations.

The first way to diagnose the back is to observe the overall feeling from it. Is it tense and rigid or relaxed and loose? Observe the muscles and the curves of the back, paying attention to whether one side is higher than the other. Notice any obvious areas of holding. When you have done this, gently touch each of the diagnostic areas in turn and see if the quality of the energy feels any different underneath your hand. Take into account that the bony structures will feel hard and the muscle softer. You are not trying to feel the structures and their nature, but rather whether they are full of or lacking in energy.

With both back and hara diagnoses you can try observing *kyo* and *jitsu*, but do not spend too much time figuring out

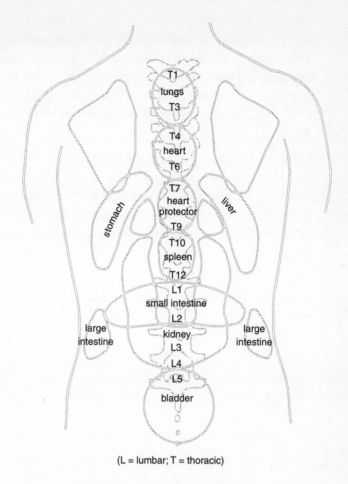

T1
lungs
T3

T4
heart
T6

T7
heart
protector
T9

T10
spleen
T12
L1
small intestine
L2
kidney
L3
L4
L5
bladder

stomach

liver

large
intestine

large
intestine

(L = lumbar; T = thoracic)

Illustration 3: Back Diagnosis Areas

what is going on. The more you dwell on what you are feeling, the more your mind steps in and draws some "logical" conclusion rather than the diagnosis being something that comes from a more intuitive level.

USING THE FIVE ELEMENTS IN DIAGNOSIS

Having looked at and experienced the various qualities expressed by the meridians, they can be seen in the context of the five elements. Each pair of the meridians is associated with one of the five elements — fire, earth, metal, water or wood. It is therefore possible to see a *kyo* lung meridian as a deficiency in the metal element. If the metal energy is depleted, the next part of the creative cycle — that is, water (kidneys) — will not receive sufficient energy to function with ease and it too will reflect a depletion of *kyo* to some degree.

In the control cycle (see Chapter Four) you can see that fire controls metal and metal in turn controls wood; therefore a deficiency or weakness in the fire element (heart) could be the cause of the metal (lung) deficiency. A *kyo* lung can lead to a disfunction of wood (liver) energy. And so the cycle continues with one element always affecting another.

Through looking, listening and touching you will develop a feeling for where in the five-element cycle the person you are treating fits, and so you will often see more clearly the underlying cause for their presenting condition.

7

GIVING A SHIATSU TREATMENT

WHO CAN GIVE A SHIATSU?

The effectiveness of a shiatsu treatment depends
on the attitude, proficiency and attunement of the
practitioner to the receiver. Anyone can give such
a treatment, provided that some basic guidelines
are followed:

- clear intention — be clear about what you
  want to do and why

- mindfulness — have your mind fully set on
  what you are doing

- no expectations — try not to have expectations of what you want to achieve

- centered — be centered or grounded before
  you start (see Chapter Eight on breathing)

- work from your *hara* (your lower abdomen)

- always use two hands, to maintain continuity,
  and keep your shoulders relaxed

- continuity — keep up a continuous flow once
  you have started

- breathing — make sure your breath is coming from the lower abdomen

- be guided by intuition, not intellect

- slow, gradual pressure when you make contact, increasing the pressure gradually while exhaling

The receiver should not experience marked discomfort, and you should not end up exhausted having given a shiatsu treatment.

When Shiatsu Massage Should Not be Applied

There are certain conditions for which it is not advisable to use shiatsu. These include:

- appendicitis (or any internal inflammation)

- cancer (except by an experienced practitioner)

- cirrhosis of the liver

- contagious disease

- fever (high)

- fractured bones

- heart disorders (severe)

- immediately after surgery

- intestinal obstruction

- peritonitis

- pyelitis

Use your discretion. If an elderly person asks for a treatment, for example, it may be necessary to do a more limited shiatsu while she sits on a chair or lies on a bed.

Pregnancy

It is safest not to give any shiatsu for the first three months of pregnancy, as some points may stimulate the uterus to contract. After the first trimester, shiatsu should only be given to the upper half of the body, down as far as the buttocks since some activation of the leg meridians could bring on early labor. The points of elimination on the large intestine meridian should never be used during pregnancy. Spleen 6 point should always be avoided.

PREPARATION OF THE TREATMENT ROOM

Have two comfortable chairs in the room so that you can sit and chat with your partner before you start and after you finish the treatment. Keep the room warm because your partner will cool down considerably once she relaxes, and have an extra blanket handy in case she gets cold. Have as few distractions as possible — perhaps only a little relaxing music. Make sure that the futon or blankets you are using for lying on are thick enough and have clean covers. If there are any odors around that may cause a distraction, burn a little incense or aromatic oils in a burner.

Make sure that your partner knows not to eat a heavy meal within the hour before the treatment. It is most comfortable if both giver and receiver wear loose comfortable clothes — preferably cotton. Your own nails need to be short, and remove all jewelry.

SHIATSU TECHNIQUES

PALMING/LEANING

This technique is commonly used to work on the different meridians and is frequently used before doing a more specific technique, such as pressing with thumbs (see Illustration 4).

Practice first on a bath towel rolled up into a sausage shape. Kneel on the floor; then put your palms on the towel in front of you and lean on them. At first, put as much pressure as you can on your palms by really pushing. Notice how much effort this requires and how tired you would feel after half

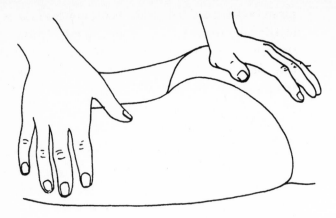

Illustration 4: Pressing with Thumbs

an hour. Next, move your body away from the towel a little and rest your palms on the towel. Very slowly, shift your body weight from your knees to your palms. Rest there for five to ten seconds. See how much more comfortable it is to lean with your body weight rather than press with force — shiatsu should never involve force.

Now find a willing subject and practice these two different ways of palming and see which feels the most comfortable for both you and your partner.

When leaning, imagine that the origin of the energy is in your *hara* and that you are extending this energy outward to your partner through your hands and arms. If you want to use this technique on a particular meridian, use the heel of the hand because you can be a little more specific.

PRESSING WITH THUMBS

This technique is used to locate *tsubos* (pressure points) and meridians more specifically and also to encourage energy into a *kyo* area. Use the ball or pad of the thumb rather than the tip (see Illustration 4).

As with palming, first place your thumb on the towel and press very hard into it. Feel how uncomfortable this is. Next, move back a little and place your thumb on the towel and slowly lean some weight on to it, gradually increasing the pressure. You should notice that even when a considerable amount of your body weight is on your thumb it is not as uncomfortable as when you pressed hard into the towel with muscle force. Always apply the thumb pressure steadily and slowly — do not jiggle or rotate it. If you press very hard and fast, the receiver will get a shock and will usually react by tensing up muscles and expecting more discomfort. This will prevent the body from really letting go and relaxing — the opposite effect to what you desire. Imagine you are pressing through seven layers of muscle before you meet resistance. When you meet resistance, hold the thumb in place for two to three seconds and then release it.

When using the pressing technique, choose points along a meridian that are approximately 4 to 6 inches apart. Hold each point for four to five seconds, release the pressure and move to the next one. If a point seems very lifeless or *kyo*, repeat this pressing and holding a few times.

Practice these two on your friend and ask which felt the most comfortable and comforting. The slow pressing should have been best.

Some other techniques that are used less frequently in this routine are outlined below.

HOLDING

This is usually used on a very *kyo* area, which can be very sensitive. The hand is just held over the area and left until some change is felt. If nothing is felt after two or three minutes, move on to another part of the body and perhaps return to this area later.

KNEADING

This motion is like kneading dough, using thumbs and fingers or the whole hand, and is used to increase circulation to an area and to loosen stiffness. It is applied mainly to the neck and shoulders and around stiff joints. The idea is to work deep into the muscles with firm movements.

STRETCHING

This is used to stretch muscles and tendons in order to increase flexibility and also to relax the muscles (see Illustration 5). The stretch should be done slowly and carefully and always on the exhalation.

TAPPING, CLAPPING, PUMMELING

This is a stimulating technique that helps to disperse stiffness. Either the fingertips, the side of the palm of the hand or the fists are used to execute quick, repetitive movements on a part of the body. Your wrists need to be very loose.

RUBBING

This technique is second nature to most of us. As used in shiatsu, it is no different to what we instinctively do to rub soreness or stiffness away. It helps to improve blood flow, relieves fatigue and warms the body.

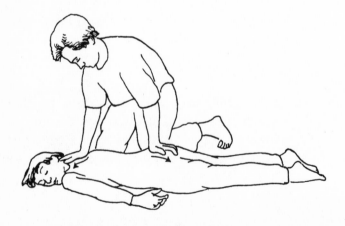

Illustration 5: Stretching the Back

MOTHER HAND

You need to keep both hands in contact with the body all the time — one is called the mother hand and the other the working hand. The mother hand is the stationary hand (usually) and its function is to give support to the client while the other hand is busy. The mother hand sits quietly observing and listening and often picks up the most reactions. In the beginning, the tendency is to forget about the mother hand because it is apparently inactive. Try to keep your awareness on *both* hands.

WORKING FROM HARA

The *hara* is the lower abdomen, the area below the ribs and above the pelvis, the center of which is the umbilicus. When giving a shiatsu treatment, keep in contact with your *hara*, the physical center of your body. This contact encourages a feeling of being grounded and connected with yourself and what is around you. By practicing lower abdominal breathing, you are directing energy to the *hara* and so encouraging this feeling of being centered.

Think of your *hara* as a spotlight shining on whatever you are doing. The *hara* should face whatever part of the body you are working on, so you must constantly adjust your position relative to your partner. By working like this, you will have greater balance and focus.

LEARNING TO GIVE SHIATSU

The best way to learn shiatsu is in a hands-on situation where it is easiest to pick up a feeling for it. If it is not possible to attend classes, however, careful study from a book is adequate if accompanied by a lot of practice. If you are learning from a book, it is important to read and practice from Chapter Eight so that you develop skills that will encourage you to focus, become more aware and sensitive.

BASIC SHIATSU ROUTINE

BACK SHIATSU

This routine is suitable for use on anyone who can lie on the floor with ease, but not for people with severe breathing problems or a bad heart condition. It is easiest to work if your partner is lying with her face to one side and hands out to the side. If this is not comfortable, try having her hands under her head. In this routine, you are working on the bladder meridian, which is a good place to diagnose the overall condition of the body. Along this meridian are the *yu* (or associated) points, all of which correspond to internal organs and functions.

1. Ask your partner to lie face down on the mat. Start by sitting on her left hand side in the *seiza* position, i.e. kneeling down and sitting back on your heels. Place your right hand on the lower back and the left hand on the upper back. Allow one or two minutes to make a connection with your partner by relaxing and breathing slowly from your lower abdomen. Encourage your partner to close her eyes and focus on her own breathing. Glance over the body to see if there are any obvious tensions in the muscles and if there are, encourage relaxation in these areas.

2. Remind yourself of your intentions in giving this treatment and remain mindful and focused on what you are doing.

3. Gently increase the pressure from your right hand on the lower back and start to rock the back. Allow the rocking movement to gather its own momentum, continuing for up to a minute. Her body should become loose and floppy.

4. Slow down the movement and get up on your right knee. Place your left foot on the floor beside your partner's head.

5. Place your left hand on the top of the back of the spine, just below the neck, fingers facing toward the head. Place your right hand on the lower back, fingers facing the opposite way (see Illustration 5). As your partner exhales, press your hands downward and away from each other as though you were trying to make the back two inches longer. Hold this for five to six seconds and repeat three times. This gives the spine a good stretch.

6. Keep your body in the same position as for the previous technique and place both palms like wings on either side of the spine. As your partner exhales, gradually lean your weight on to your hands, keeping your elbows straight. Make sure that the pressure is one of leaning and not pushing. Hold for three to four seconds and relax. You should find five or six places to do this, moving down along the back. Move your own body back down toward your partner's feet as your hands move down the back. When you come to the sacrum (the triangular bone at the end of the spine), hold for ten seconds. Repeat three times.

7. Place your hands over one another like a cross and put them over the lower back. Gently lean your weight on to them and hold for ten seconds. This can feel very good for someone with a weak lower back, although it is *not* suitable for someone with severe backache.

8. Locate the vertebrae of the spine with your left hand as your right hand stays on the lower back. Trace the vertebrae down to the lower back.

9. With the outside edges of the palms of your hands, rub vigorously up and down either side of the spine as though trying to warm up your partner. As one hand goes up one side of the back, the other goes down.

10. Knead the upper back and the shoulders, paying particular attention to the area between the spine and shoulder blades. Squeeze and knead deep into these areas with your thumbs.

11. Place your thumbs eleven and a half thumb widths on either side of the top of the spine. With the pads of the thumbs in contact with the back, slowly let your thumbs sink into the back and hold for four or five seconds. Make sure that your arms are straight yet relaxed and your thumbs perpendicular to the skin. Sink in gradually — imagine you are sinking through seven layers of muscle before you meet resistance (see Illustration 6). Move your thumbs a little farther down the back and repeat, sinking in, holding and releasing. As you continue all the way down the spine, see if you can notice any difference between the various places you come in contact with.

By working like this down the bladder meridian you are contacting all the nerve bundles that radiate out from the spine, stimulating various functions in the body. You are also making contact with the *yu* points of energy.

Now move to the level of your partner's hips.

12. Place your left hand on the lower back. Draw an imaginary line down the center of the back of the leg. With

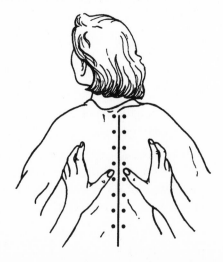

Illustration 6: Pressing Down Bladder Meridian
on Back with Thumbs

your right hand, palm across the buttocks and down the center of the back of the left leg, leaning, holding and releasing. Try to connect with what is going on — is the leg tense, relaxed, sensitive?

13. Press with your thumb down this same area from the buttocks to the toes. Remember to find the point first, then press slowly in, hold and release.

(Take care around the calves, as this area is particularly sensitive.) When you reach the Achilles' tendon, pinch the area between the tendon and the ankle bones and continue a pinching movement down the outside of the foot until you reach the little toe. Make sure that you keep one hand stable, preferably on the sacrum, and focus on your breathing. (If your partner is a lot taller than you, you may have to move your mother hand down the leg a little as you move.)

Repeat on the other leg.

14. Then, kneel at your partner's feet and hold up the ankles. With a firm grip, pull the legs toward you as you lean back, as though trying to add two inches to your partner's height.

15. Bend the legs at the knee and push the feet toward the buttocks. Hold and then relax. Repeat three times.

16. Staying on your partner's left side, slide the left knee and foot outward so that the knee is almost at right angles to the body (see Illustration 7). This is a stretch for the gall bladder meridian. Place yourself at your partner's legs. Keep your right hand on the lower back. With your left hand, follow the same technique and sequence of first palming and then pressing with the thumb down the meridian. Palm down the center of the side of the leg first and then press all the way down, finishing up at the fourth toe. Put the leg back in the starting position.

Repeat the same sequence on the other leg.

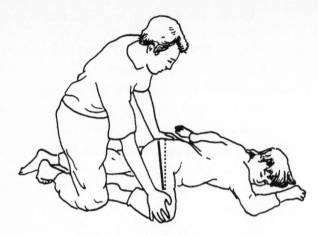

Illustration 7: Gall Bladder Stretch

Straighten your partner's legs. With loose fists, tap all over the back, buttocks and thighs. You can also do this tapping with the outside edge of the palm of your hand. Try to do it rhythmically, with loose, floppy wrists.

Finish the back by sitting beside your partner with both hands on her back. Listen to what is going on, and relax yourself, focusing on your breath.

NECK AND SHOULDER SHIATSU

Ask your partner to kneel, if possible with buttocks on heels (in the seiza position). If this position is not comfortable, do this technique with your partner sitting on a chair.

1.   If she is on a chair, her feet should be on the floor and not crossed. Encourage her to close her eyes because this shuts out visual stimuli. Encourage her to focus on her breath, allowing it to get deeper and slower. Rub your hands together vigorously and place them on your partner's shoulders. Wait and listen for a short while with your hands on her shoulders. See if you can feel a connection between you and your partner — is she tense, worried, sad, joyful? Look out for any obvious tension; if there is any, encourage her to let it go.

2. Relax your own shoulders and knead the muscles at the back of her shoulders with your thumbs. Grip your fingers around the top of the shoulders for stability. Work deeply into the muscles and tissues all around the area of muscle between the spine in the center and the shoulder blades. Use a circular rather than a simple pressing and holding movement.

3. Squeeze along the top of the shoulders with the thumbs and fingers, starting at the neck and working out toward the edge of the shoulders.

4. Place your palms under her elbows. Ask your client to inhale while you raise the elbows up so that the shoulders are up around her ears. Ask her to hold her breath for five seconds and then exhale. As the exhalation is completed, allow the shoulders to flop down. Repeat three times.

5. Stand on the left side of your partner. Hold her forehead with your left hand. With your right thumb on one side of the neck and fingers on the other side, knead down the back of the neck, starting where the head meets the neck and finishing where the neck meets the shoulders (see Illustration 8). Your movements should be slow,

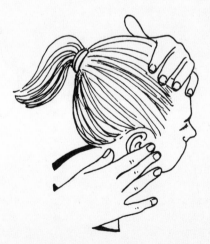

Illustration 8: Thumbing the Neck

deliberate and deep. This area holds a lot of tension and usually needs considerable attention. Massage deep into the areas where you feel the most tension. Make sure that you do not forget about the hand supporting her forehead — do not let it squeeze too hard or cover the eyes.

6. Secure the neck by gripping it firmly with your right hand. With your left hand on the top of the head, rotate it slowly in a wide circle, three times one way, and three times the other way. You may hear a lot of cracks and creaks. Encourage your partner to relax and let you do the rotating.

7. With your left hand again on the forehead, use your right thumb to locate the ridge under the skull around the hairline (see Illustration 9). Keeping your thumb on the hairline, move it to the center of the back of the skull, where you will feel a little depression. Press your thumb into the depression, upward and inward, gradually increasing the pressure until you feel resistance.

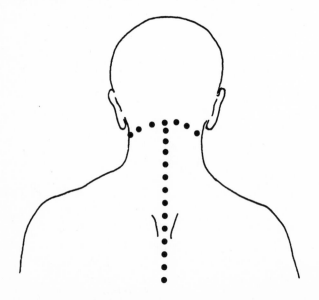

Illustration 9: Neck and Shoulder Shiatsu

Hold for five seconds and then release. Repeat three times. Use the hand on the forehead to steady the head and to give counter pressure.

8. Move your thumb one inch in the direction of the left ear, keeping your thumb on the hairline. Press upward and inward very gradually as before, and hold for five seconds. Continue this until you reach the hard bone behind the left ear. If you find a painful point, spend more time on it, pressing more gently and holding a little longer. Repeat from the center depression to the ear three times.

9. Move to the other side of your partner and repeat 8 on the other side.

10. Move to the back of your partner again. Press the points on the top of the shoulders. Place your thumbs on top of the shoulders in the corner where the neck joins the shoulder. Position the thumb so that it is pointing downward, as though you were pressing through the shoulder to the floor. With both thumbs simultaneously sink into the top of the shoulders, increasing the pressure until you meet resistance; then hold for five seconds and release. Move your thumbs one inch out toward the edge of the shoulder and press, hold and release again. Continue this slowly until you reach the outside edge of the shoulder where you feel the muscle disappearing. Make sure that your own shoulders are relaxed.

The following exercise is a neck stretch.

11. Hold your right hand on your partner's right shoulder and hold the right side of her head with your left hand. Inhale. As she exhales, push the shoulder down and gently move the head toward the left. Hold for eight seconds and relax. Repeat three times. Move to the other side and repeat again, this time moving the head to the right.

12. With the side of the palm of your hands, stimulate the top of the shoulders and the top of the back with a vigorous clapping movement.

13. Ask your partner to join her hands behind her head. Take her elbows in the palms of your hands and ask her to inhale. As she exhales, pull her shoulders toward you and hold for a few seconds. Then relax and repeat. This is a very good stretch for anyone with chest complaints, depression and rounded shoulders.

14. Finish off by resting your hands gently on the top of the shoulders.

SHIATSU WHILE LYING ON THE BACK

Ask your partner to lie on her back in a comfortable position. Make sure she is relaxed and warm, with her hands at her side and palms facing upward.

1. Lift her knees up, bend the legs and push the knees toward the chest. Ask her to inhale, and on the exhalation, press her knees to the chest and hold this stretch for ten seconds. Repeat three times.

2. Place the legs in the outstretched position again and come to your partner's right side. Take the right leg and cross it over the left leg, with the right foot on the outside of the left knee. Hold the right knee with your right hand and have your left hand on the right shoulder. Both inhale, and on the exhalation press the knee toward the floor while anchoring the right shoulder with your hand. Hold the stretch for ten seconds, relax and repeat twice more.

   Move to the other side and repeat three times (see Illustration 10).

   This exercise is very good for the hips and lower back, but it must be done with caution. You should only do the stretch when your partner is exhaling and must not push if there is pain or a lot of resistance. As with any

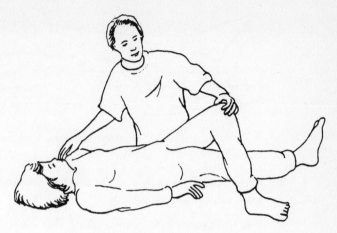

Illustration 10: Back and Hip Stretch

stretch, for the exercise to be of use you need to be sensitive but at the same time firm.

3.   Move your partner's right arm out of the way and sit close to her in the *seiza* position, facing toward her head.

4.   Place your right hand on her lower abdomen and watch to see if the breath is reaching this area. If the breath appears to be higher up in the chest, encourage her to breathe into the lower abdomen, gently pushing your hand up as she inhales and letting it fall as she exhales. Attend to the breath until it becomes slow and deep in the abdomen.

STOMACH MERIDIAN

Locate this meridian before you work on it and do a stretch to expose it and bring it to the surface.

1.   Turn a little so that you are facing perpendicular to your partner. Keep your left knee on the floor and put your right foot close to your partner's right foot. Take the foot and press it toward the floor. At the same time, hold the top of the thigh as though stretching a line all the way down the center of the leg (see Illustration 11).

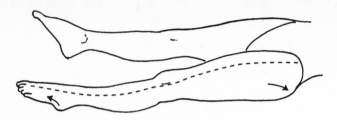

Illustration 11: Stomach Meridian Stretch

2. Palm down the center of the thigh from the top to the knee, slowly and mindfully.

3. Use the pressing technique along this same line to the knee. The stomach meridian runs down the outside of the leg from the side of the knee, parallel to the shin bone, over the front of the ankle to the second toe.

4. Press along this line, keeping your thumb perpendicular to the skin so that you are pressing straight inward and not at an angle. Make sure that you find a point, gradually increase the pressure, hold and then release it.

    Pay particular attention to a *tsubo* — stomach 36 — that is located four finger widths below the bottom of the knee cap and one thumb width out from the shin bone. This is one of the important *tsubos* in the body and is useful for digestive problems, tiredness and leg pains.

Leg Rotation

5. Position yourself at your partner's right knee, facing her head. With your right knee on the floor and left foot at the level of your partner's hips, bend her knee; hold the right foot with your right hand and her knee with your left hand. Push the knee toward the chest. Then, with a rotating swing, move it outward to your left in an counter-clockwise direction to stretch the groin and upper leg. Repeat this circular stretch for four or five rotations in an counter-clockwise direction and then the same number of times in a clockwise direction.

Repeat this on the other side before you work on the left stomach meridian.

Repeat 1, 2, 3, 4 and 5 on the other side.

When you have completed the left side, come down to the feet and sit in the *seiza* position. Pick up the left foot and place it in your lap. Hold the heel in your left palm, and with your right hand rotate the foot three times one way and three times the other way. Do the maximum stretch possible all the time. You may hear cracks and creaks as you rotate the limbs — these are reasonably common.

Repeat this on the right foot.

SPLEEN MERIDIAN AND SPLEEN STRETCH

The spleen meridian runs from the big toe around the top of the ankle bone through an important *tsubo* (spleen 6), situated four finger widths above the inside ankle bone, just behind the shin bone. It then travels up the inside of the leg behind the shin bone, through the side of the knee over the inside of the front of the thigh.

Move up the body (on the right side) so that you are level with your partner's right knee. Place her right foot at the left ankle so that the right knee falls outward toward you.

1. Press the right knee toward the floor while steadying the left hip on the floor with your left hand. This is stretching the spleen meridian. Hold it for five seconds and release (see Illustration 12). Repeat three times. This stretch allows the meridian to be exposed so that it is easier to work on.

2. Put your knees under your partner's bent knee for support, while you palm up the spleen meridian from the big toe as far as the knee. Keep your left hand on the *hara* and see if there is any reaction in this area while you are working. Then thumb this three times, paying particular attention to the *tsubo* spleen 6. This is good

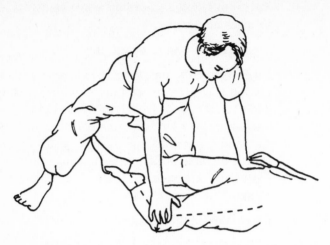

Illustration 12: Spleen Meridian and Spleen Stretch

for menstrual and digestive problems plus insomnia. **Note:** *Do not press this point if the client is pregnant.*

3.   When you reach the knee, palm up the inside of the thigh. Then press from the knee to the top of the thigh three times.

Remember that throughout the treatment your stationary hand is there on the *hara* to listen to what is going on and to be a comfort to your partner.

LIVER MERIDIAN STRETCH

The liver meridian runs from the inside of the big toe between the first and second toes, over the front of the foot and in front of the ankle bone, through *tsubo* spleen 6. It then crosses the spleen meridian and goes on the inside of the lower leg to the knee and then parallel to the spleen meridian up the inner thigh.

1.   Remain in the same position as above. Take the right knee in your right hand and press it toward the chest. Hold on the exhalation for ten seconds. Repeat three times.

2. To stretch the liver meridian, place the right foot beside the opposite knee and let the right knee fall outward toward you. Again with your left hand on the left hip, hold it down and put pressure on the right knee, pressing it gently toward the floor. Hold the stretch for five seconds and repeat three times. The stretch will vary in different people, depending on their flexibility.

3. Palm from the ankle to the knee, keeping parallel to the shin bone. Continue to palm from the knee up the center of the inside of the thigh to the top of the thigh.

4. Press from the ankle to the top of the inner thigh.

5. Go to the end of your partner's body and kneel at her feet. Pick up both legs and swing them from side to side a few times in a loose movement.

Go to the left side of your partner and repeat the sequence for both the spleen and liver meridians.

HARA SHIATSU

In Western anatomy, the *hara* is the area enclosed by a line drawn around the outside of the abdomen, starting at the top of the rib cage and following in a clockwise direction under the ribs around the side to the pelvis, along the pelvic bone to the other side and up to the rib cage (see Illustration 2). The *hara* is considered a very important area in Japanese life. It is understood to be the center of energy and balance, where energy is stored and generated for use. A healthy *hara* indicates overall good health and the reverse is also true. The Japanese expression to commit hara kiri means to cut out the *hara*. This is a ritual form of suicide where a knife is put through the *hara*. In a less literal sense, it describes someone willing to take responsibility for their actions.

In shiatsu, the *hara* is used as an area for diagnosis. It is the area where the overall state of the body and its functions can be assessed. All the digestive and female reproductive organs are in the *hara* area, even if only on the border. It is here that food is converted into energy, so the correct functioning of the *hara* is vital to good *ki* production.

The *hara* is very sensitive, as it is not protected by bony structures and therefore needs to be treated with great care. If the receiver is feeling very vulnerable, it can be good just to hold this area gently. A lot of tension can be held here, and often it is not until a *hara* massage is given that such tension is recognized. During a treatment, a lot of gurgling and rumbling can be felt, which is a sign of letting go and relaxing.

HARA MASSAGE ROUTINE

1. Sit in the *seiza* position on the right side of your partner, facing toward her.

2. Place your right hand over her *tanden* area (four fingers below the navel). Place the other hand underneath the breast bone. Gently rest your hands here and observe your partner to see that the breath is slow and in the lower abdomen. Sometimes you may feel a strong pulse beating here — don't worry, it just means that your partner is still alive! This pulse is the largest artery in the body — the aorta — feeding the lower part of the body with blood.

3. Place one hand over the other and slowly let them circle around the border of the *hara* three or four times in a clockwise direction.

4. This next movement is known as "rocking the *hara*." Turn so that you are facing your partner's *hara*. Place your hands on top of each other on the *hara* so that they are facing away from you. Pull the abdomen toward you with your finger tips and then push it away using the heels of your hand. This technique should not just move the surface but the muscles and also the organs below. (**Note:** For this reason, it is not advisable to do it right after a meal — wait for about an hour.) Repeat this movement for ten strokes.

5. Using four fingers of the right hand, gently press into the solar plexus, just below the center of the rib cage. Then move your hand to your right and press along the underside of the rib cage. Continue tracing the abdomen clockwise down to the hip bone, along the pelvis, around to the other hip bone and up to the rib cage again. This pressing movement should be gentle. Keep one hand stationary on the *hara* in a place where you are not touching with your other hand. Repeat three times.

6. "Lifting the *hara*" is a technique that helps to release any remaining tension in the abdomen. Place your hands underneath the *hara* so that your fingers are in contact with the spine and as though you are making a sling to lift your partner with. Lift up the back slowly from underneath as your partner exhales, and give your hands a gentle shake while lowering the back to the floor again. Repeat three times.

7. Finish by holding one hand underneath the *hara* and the other on top so that the *hara* is like a sandwich. Hold here as long as it feels comfortable. This is very relaxing.

While working on the *hara*, you will notice that some areas are quite hard and others soft — or that some areas are full (*jitsu*) and others empty (*kyo*). Through these observations, diagnosis can be made and appropriate treatment can follow. Picking up subtle differences develops with practice. If you do find a particular area that is remarkable in having too much energy or too little, refer back to Illustration 2. If you find a very *kyo* area, hold it gently for two to three minutes.

Shiatsu on the Arm Meridians

1. Stay on the right side of your partner. Place your right knee at the level of your partner's waist and your left foot at her shoulder. Put one palm on each of your partner's shoulders and lean your body weight forward on to the shoulders, keeping your arms straight yet relaxed. Repeat three times.

2. Move down so that you are level with your partner's waist. Move the right arm away from the body with the palm facing upward. Hold your right hand on the right shoulder, and with your left hand palm down the inside of the arm three times (see Illustration 13).

The following will cover the three meridians on the inside of the arm — the lung, the heart governor and the heart. Draw three imaginary lines from the shoulder to the fingers, all running parallel to each other. These are the lung (running to the thumb); the heart constrictor (running down the center of the arm to the middle finger); and the heart (which runs close to the inside edge of the arm to the inside of the little finger).

3. Press from the top of the shoulder to the thumb three times, choosing a point to press, sinking in, holding and then releasing. This is the lung meridian. An important point on this meridian is lung 1. It is situated below the middle of the collar bone, in the space between the first and second ribs. Press this three times, holding for five seconds each time.

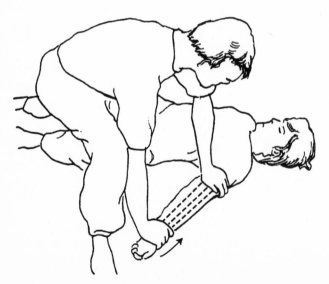

Illustration 13: Palming Arms Meridian

4. Press down the center of the arm from the shoulder to the middle finger to work on the heart constrictor meridian. An important *tsubo* is heart constrictor 6, which is located two inches above the wrist fold, in between the two tendons. This is useful for someone with palpitations. Press and hold for five seconds. Repeat three times. Heart constrictor 8 is in the center of the palm of the hand, and can be pressed as above. This technique is useful for those suffering from exhaustion.

5. To work on the heart meridian, bend the arm so that the hand is above the head (see Illustration 14). In this position the heart meridian is exposed and you can work on it more easily. If the arm does not rest easily on the floor, place a blanket or your knee under it. Work from the inside of the armpit along the bottom edge of the arm and down to the inside of the little finger. Return the hand to the side of the body.

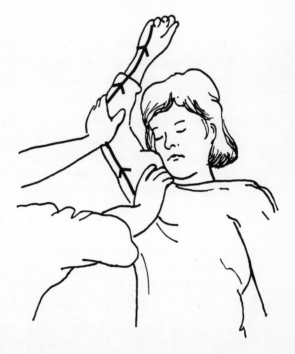

Illustration 14: Heart Meridian Stretch

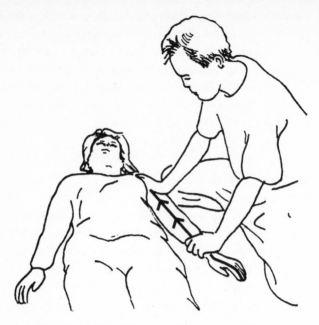

Illustration 15: Shiatsu on All Arm Meridians

6. Massage the hand by opening up the palm and kneading into the muscles. Massage all the fingers, pulling them and rotating them in turn.

7. Turn the hand so that the palm is facing down. Pull the arm toward you and shake it. Place your right hand on the shoulder, and with your left hand palm from the fingers up to the shoulder (see Illustration 15). This technique covers all three meridians on this side of the arm.

8. Again, draw three imaginary lines parallel to one another going up the arm: one from the thumb to the shoulder — the large intestine meridian; one up the center of the arm from the ring finger — the triple heater; and one from the little finger up the outside edge of the arm — the small intestine meridian.

9. Thumb the large intestine meridian from the index finger to the shoulder three times. The most important point on this meridian is large intestine 4, which is locat-

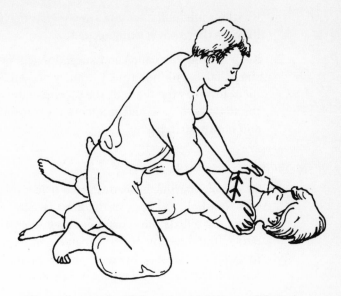

Illustration 16: Small Intestine Meridian and Stretch

ed in the web between the thumb and first finger. This point is useful for general health and for treating intestinal problems, facial pain and toothache. Press and hold for ten seconds. Repeat three times.

10. Thumb the triple heater meridian from the ring finger up the center of the arm to the shoulder.

11. Thumb the small intestine meridian by starting at the little finger and working along the outside of the hand, along the outside edge of the ulnar bone to the elbow (see Illustration 16). It is then easiest to locate it if the arm is bent across the chest, exposing the underneath part of the upper arm. Thumb along the center of the triceps muscle on the under part of the arm, up to the shoulder.

ARM STRETCH

1. Stand behind your partner's head. Take both her hands in your hands and raise them up so that they are at right angles to her body. First pull one upward then the other.

Rhythmically pull alternate arms so that the upper body looks as though it is being rocked.

2. Keep holding the hands and kneel down at her head. As she exhales, pull her arms toward you, gently lowering them towards the floor. In some people, the arms reach the floor with ease and in others they are much stiffer and hardly stretch at all.

NECK SHIATSU IN THE LYING POSITION

1. Sit at your partner's head. Put your feet on her shoulders and hold the back of the head (where it meets the neck). On exhalation, push your feet against her shoulders in the direction of her feet and gently pull her head toward you. Most of the force should be in the feet, not on the head. Relax and repeat three times.

2. Turn her face to the left and put one hand on the back of her head and the other on the right shoulder. On the exhalation, push the shoulder downward while very gently encouraging the head to the left. Relax and repeat three times. Repeat on the other side.

3. Turn the face to the left. With your right thumb, massage around the ridge at the base of the head around the hairline. Work from the ear to the center of the back of the head. Turn the head and do the same on the other side. (Use the same technique as for neck and shoulder shiatsu — see page 60.)

4. Massage the back of the neck by rubbing and kneading the neck with your finger tips, starting from the base of the neck and working up toward the head.

FACE SHIATSU

1. Sit in the *seiza* position at your partner's head, or if it is more comfortable, sit at her head with your legs out to either side.

2. Place your hands on either side of her face and allow the warmth of your hands to penetrate her face.

3. Place your thumbs on top of one another over the "third eye" — the spot at the top of the nose between the eyebrows. Gently increase the pressure, hold for five to six seconds, then release. Repeat three times.

4. Place one thumb on either side of the third eye on the ridges over the eyes. Press slowly and gradually, hold for five to six seconds and release. Repeat this until you reach the end of the rim of the eye socket.

5. Return your thumbs to the center again, but move them up a little toward the middle of the forehead. Again, work out toward the temples, pressing, holding and releasing.

6. When you reach the temples, massage them with slow, deliberate circular movements.

7. Place your thumbs on the side of the nose and press across the lower rims of the eye sockets.

8. Put your middle fingers on the joints of the jaw in front of the ears. You can locate these points by asking your partner to open and close her mouth. Massage the joint with your fingers. This can be very painful because the jaw often seems to hold a lot of tension.

9. Work your way down the lower jaw with your thumbs and fingers in a pinching movement. Start at the joint you were working on, and finish off at the rounded end of the chin.

10. Massage the scalp by using all your finger tips, working in a circular motion around the scalp.

11. Finish by holding her face between your hands again, for two to three minutes. Silently wish your partner well.

8

PRACTICES TO ENCOURAGE STABILITY OF MIND AND BODY

Giving shiatsu massage requires concentration and focus, qualities that can be enhanced through meditation, awareness exercises, yoga-style stretching exercises and appropriate nutrition. Shiatsu is best seen in the context of overall lifestyle, and a treatment is of most benefit when supported by appropriate adjustments in diet, lifestyle, exercise and thinking, both on the part of the practitioner and partner.

Developing an awareness of your breathing is a useful starting point.

BREATHING

Most meditation practices, yoga and the martial arts encourage breathing from the lower abdomen, or *hara*. Focusing attention on this area harmonizes the body, mind, emotions and spirit, helping us to feel more grounded. Breathing is synonymous with being alive. If we stop breathing we stop living, and if we breathe well we can increase our vitality and stability.

Correct breathing leads to:

- good exchange of oxygen and carbon dioxide in all the cells
- better management of stress
- better lymph drainage
- improved circulation
- feeling connected and a sense of well-being
- feeling grounded or centered
- feeling relaxed

BREATHING EXERCISES

Close your eyes and observe how you breathe. Is your breath caught up in your chest or does it go deep down into your abdomen?

PRACTICE EXERCISE

1. Lie on the ground or sit in a position where your spine is straight.

2. Tense all the muscles in your body completely as you inhale. Concentrate on the tension and hold tight for eight to ten seconds. Gradually let the muscles go as you exhale and feel the contrast. Try to let go and relax totally. Repeat two to three times.

3. Exhale completely.

4. To check whether you are breathing into your lower abdomen, place one hand on your chest and the other on the abdomen below the navel.

5. Inhale and see which hand moves the most. If your breathing is efficient, the lower hand should move the most.

To ensure that you have understood lower abdominal breathing:

6.   Inhale very, very slowly, allowing the breath to enter effortlessly through your nose. At the same time, push out your abdomen as though you were blowing up a balloon in your belly. Move your chest as little as possible.

7.   After your abdomen is stretched, expand your chest with air. This fills up the middle part of your lungs. Hold the breath for about five seconds and then slowly begin to exhale. As you do so, let your abdomen fall and relax. Repeat this for twenty breaths. Focus your attention on the movement of your abdomen as you inhale and exhale.

As you continue to do this regularly, you will have to put less effort into expanding your abdomen — your breath will do that for you. After a while, lower abdominal breathing will become second nature. If you practice it each day while lying down, it will become easier to do it even when going about routine tasks in the house, at work or in the street. Become aware of when your breath gets caught up in your chest. When this happens, consciously drop your shoulders and place a hand on your lower abdomen and breathe into this area, allowing your abdomen to expand. Then exhale, with a feeling of letting go.

DEVELOPING MINDFULNESS

In order to gain more insight into what we are doing and why, it is important to develop a quality of mindfulness. Increased awareness brings greater equanimity into our lives. In shiatsu practice, we need to focus on what we are doing and to have a keen awareness of the interaction between ourselves and our partner, of feelings and reactions. Mindfulness helps to encourage this and to focus our attention directly on the task at hand.

Mindfulness is about developing a continuous awareness of all the tasks we do and the thoughts we have during the course of a normal day. We should pay the most attention to what we do automatically — like drinking a cup of tea, going to the lavatory, washing the dishes, running up and down stairs. So often we do not have our minds on what we are doing — our bodies are doing one thing and our minds are on a totally different tack, which creates disharmony. In order to turn off our "automatic pilot," we need to develop more awareness of what we are doing, to do things more slowly so that we can see each part of the routine action more clearly. Try doing tasks as though for the first time, so that they require your full concentration.

How often do you get to the top of the stairs and do not remember why you went up there in the first place? Have you ever overslept for ten minutes, got up in a rush and spent the rest of the day catching up? If we become conscious of each change and reaction that takes place in the body, we can see things as they arise rather than after they have happened.

EXERCISE IN MINDFULNESS

It is essential for a shiatsu practitioner to practice exercises in mindfulness. Choose something you do without thinking regularly during the day — such as making a cup of coffee. Start by making a resolution that you are going to follow through this exercise without interruptions. Do it with careful attention, very slowly, and notice each part of the task as you do it. See how easy it is to speed up again as you forget that you are trying to do it slowly!

Take the kettle and fill it with water, turning the tap on slowly, turning it off with great caution. Place the kettle back on the stove without a bump; wait for it to boil. Don't go off and do ten jobs while it comes to the boil. Take out your cup and place the coffee filter into it and very carefully pour the water onto it. Wait for it to drip for the required amount of time and then put the filter in the trash can. Walk slowly over to the refrigerator, open the door carefully, take out the milk and close the door. Walk back to the cup and pour in the milk as slowly as you can and then return it to the refrigerator.

Sit down. Wait. Pick up the cup carefully, as though it would break if you touched it forcefully. Bring the cup to your mouth very slowly. Sip the coffee and really taste it, feel the texture of it, notice the temperature of it. Place the cup down, wait, pause, pick it up again and continue like this until you have finished. Notice how often during this simple routine your mind wanders on to something else.

Be aware of:

- your impatience at the slow speed
- what it feels like to be attentive to this task
- how often your mind wanders off elsewhere

If you do this a number of times, you will recognize that we spend very little time in the present. So much of the day is spent doing things physically while the mind is somewhere else, leading to confusion, forgetfulness and a feeling of not being in control.

Other ways of developing mindfulness are to listen to ourselves and to ask:

- what am I doing?
- why am I doing it?
- do I listen well to others?

Reflect inward more frequently and check in to what is going on inside. Try to make space between tasks that you do, consciously completing one before you start the next. Finish the day by recapping what you have done during the day.

MEDITATION

The purpose of meditation is to slow down so that we can see clearly into the nature of the mind, making it possible for us to become fully present in each moment, to gain understanding of the way things truly are. It can give rise to the deep sense of calm that comes from really knowing something for yourself. In order to have peace of mind, we need to discover what is preventing us from accessing our inner peace. An uncontrolled mind can never find peace and satisfaction. Besides all the noise in our conscious minds, we also have a lot of confusion and noise in the unconscious mind. In order to create space in the mind we have to start right here.

Meditation encourages:

- our ability to focus
- calmness and equanimity
- awareness
- insight into what is going on inside us

Developing the above qualities will enhance communication between receiver and giver during a shiatsu treatment.

Meditation can be difficult for beginners because it is in complete contrast to how we normally conduct our daily lives. Many meditation techniques have a similar approach — they encourage you to focus on something specific such as the breath, a candle or a mantra (called objects of meditation). Whatever arises in the mind or body, the intention is to remain focused on the object of meditation. Thoughts will arise in the mind and sensations in the body, but rather than getting caught up with these distractions the idea is merely to observe them, not commenting, and return to the object of meditation. In time it is possible to become a passive observer of all the feelings and sensations that come and go — not attaching to them — which creates a calm acceptance of the way things are.

LEARNING TO MEDITATE

Set aside a time to meditate when you know you are not rushing to do something, so that you can give your full attention to it.

1. Use a posture that will allow your back to be straight without strain. This can be in a straight-backed chair or in a cross-legged position on the floor. Make sure that you are comfortable.

2. Allow your eyes to close.

3. Gather your attention and move it slowly down through your body, starting at your head, making sure that there is a sense of calm and relaxation as you go. If you notice areas of physical tension, try to let them go as you exhale.

4. Allow your thoughts, ideas and memories to drift in and out of the mind without following them.

5. Focus your attention on the breath and allow it to come from your lower abdomen. Notice the rise and fall of the abdomen as the breath comes in and goes out. Focus your mind on the sensation of the breath, on the movement of the abdomen, and see how difficult it is to keep your attention on this simple process. As soon as you notice that your mind has wandered, return your attention to the breath and the movement of the abdomen, using the words "in and out" or "rising and falling" as the breath comes in and goes out — this can help focus the attention more sharply.

This whole process develops mindfulness, patience and insightful understanding. At times when meditating you may feel sleepy or bored. When this happens, put more effort into your posture and the bodily sensations. With regular practice, you will begin to see your attitudes more clearly and will come to know what is useful for you and what is creating difficulties in your life. You will also begin to see how the mind habitually reacts to situations and how habits can stifle progress. Try to put aside fifteen to twenty minutes each day to meditate. If you do so for only five or ten minutes, the mind has hardly had time to slow down before you wind it up again.

The mind is like a pond full of water: if you stir up the water it looks muddy, cloudy and opaque; likewise, because we are constantly agitating it, the mind becomes cloudy and busy. If you take a glass of muddy water from the pond and let it rest on a window ledge for twenty minutes, the silt will sink to the bottom, leaving clear water. In the same way, if you sit for twenty minutes without agitating the mind, your thoughts will slow down and some clarity will emerge.

PHYSICAL EXERCISES

Giving a shiatsu treatment requires physical flexibility because you have to spend close to fifteen minutes on the floor, mainly on your knees. If you intend to give advice to others, it is always better received if there is a conviction about what you are advising, which comes from personal experience. Exercises can be a tremendous support to shiatsu treatments and to overall health.

The physical exercises that best support shiatsu by improving flexibility, concentration and the flow of *ki* energy are aikido and yoga. Aikido is a Japanese martial art, a self-defense art that encourages concentration, flexibility and strengthens and focuses *ki* energy.

YOGA

The form of yoga most compatible with shiatsu is Okido yoga. This encourages controlled breathing, meditation and physical exercise, so that we can learn how to recognize the causes of illness and imbalance and help to correct these with regular practice.

NUTRITION

It is important to become aware of the effect on the body of what we eat, and how foods affect how we feel. Over my years of shiatsu practice, I have seen that most people need some adjustments in their diet in order to support the treatment.

The most beneficial change is to cut out "extreme foods," foods that seem to have the most dramatic effect on the body. These often are, unfortunately, eaten in large quantities. The extreme effect of such foods is no longer acknowledged by the body since it becomes an accepted way of feeling for many people. An example is that of drinking strong coffee. This creates a stress-like response in the body — shaking hands, heart palpitations, dilated pupils, poor digestion and sweating. These symptoms are often accepted as "normal," because they are continuously present in some people to a greater or lesser degree.

These symptoms may be a background discomfort that can be tolerated, but stimulants create a strain on the body. It is not healthy to have a system that is constantly on the alert and under stress. By taking regular stimulants such as caffeine, sugar, alcohol, drugs and cigarettes, the body cannot relax properly. This can be a contributory factor in many stress related disorders such as ulcers, migraines, irritable bowel syndrome, psoriasis and asthma. Too many stimulants alter the mind state, thus preventing real clarity.

There are also foods that have the opposite effect, that of depressing the system. These are mainly animal foods, particularly red meat, heavy dairy foods (butter, cheese, mayonnaise, ice cream, cream) and salt. They appear to slow down the digestive system, taking a long time to pass through it. This sluggishness gives rise to constipation, bowel disorders and other symptoms such as acne, low energy, low motivation and depression. A lot of red meat slows down the body and mind. Dairy foods are also often a contributory factor in the build up of mucus in the body, particularly in the respiratory tract, the sinuses, the ears and the female reproductive organs.

In most spiritual disciplines originating from the East, there is little emphasis on animal foods, with a tendency toward vegetarianism instead.

Basic recommendations for a more balanced and nutritious diet are as follows:

FOODS TO CUT DOWN	FOODS TO INCREASE
red meat	vegetable protein
dairy foods	(lentils, beans and nuts)
sugar/cookies/cakes	whole grains
oils (except olive oil)	(brown rice, barley, millet
tea and coffee	and oats)
alcohol	fresh vegetables
refined foods	fresh fruits
cigarettes	homemade soups
	soy-based products

When some dietary changes are made there can be a reaction in the body that may seem negative. If caffeine has been taken in large quantities over a number of years, the body will experience withdrawal symptoms such as headaches and nausea. These will pass within a couple of days — be patient! If you have been used to eating a lot of animal products and either cut them down or give them up, you may get symptoms of detoxification. Your skin may temporarily become blotchy or spotty, and you may feel tired. It is worth persevering.

If you give up animal food altogether, you will have to find your protein from vegetable sources such as beans, lentils, nuts and seeds. Soy bean products are a fine way to get protein, and include tofu, tempeh, soy milk, soy sausages and burgers. You may wish just to cut down consumption of red meat to start with, and still eat chicken and fish. Take care not to overdose on chicken unless it is free range; there can be toxic residues in it. Fish is a good source of fatty acids, calcium and protein, but do not eat it too often since it may be contaminated.

To give up all sugar can be very difficult because there are hidden sugars in so many refined products — even salty ones. Beware of foods that say they are sugar free; their manufacturers often have a different way of presenting sugar, such as sucrose, maltose, dextrose, saccharin or aspartame. Some people think that honey is a good substitute for sugar, but it contains a high percentage of sugar, only some of which is naturally occurring.

Eat in moderation, and chew your food well. Try not to eat when stressed. If you are anxious about something, take a few long slow breaths before you start your meal. If you do this you will eat in a more relaxed way and your digestive system will function better. See how much of your eating is done consciously and how much is done mindlessly/anxiously and out of a need for comfort. Food should be used to nourish the physical body, not as an emotional crutch.

9

CASE STUDIES

———

Having studied shiatsu and used it on hundreds of people for more than a decade, I do not believe that it is the only answer to ill health. It certainly assists many people bring about positive change in their lives. As with any healing practice, it is difficult to separate the value of the technique as a catalyst to change from the relationship between the client and therapist. For some, it does not matter what creates the change — the important thing is that change takes place. The technique is a framework to work within in order to connect with someone and assist the process of healing. The following case studies illustrate what I mean by this.

CASE ONE: JANE

Jane is a sixty-eight-year-old woman living alone.

MEDICAL HISTORY

Jane had a hysterectomy twenty-five years ago and has constant lower back pain. She had a mild heart attack two years ago and is a borderline diabetic. With a history of anxiety and depression, Jane was on valium for twenty years until she recently changed to a milder tranquilizer.

FIRST VISIT

Jane was very distressed and quite disoriented when she arrived. She had just cried for help and someone brought her into my practice room.

Jane's sister died of breast cancer two years ago and since then Jane has been very depressed, phobic and fearful, with little peace of mind. She finds it very difficult to quieten her mind and relax — she is constantly worrying about something. Jane is overweight and has a very bloated abdomen and complains of indigestion and constipation. She also has a constant nagging pain in her back neck and shoulders. Her energy and motivation are low.

JANE'S DIET

Packet cereal and milk for breakfast followed by many slices of bread, butter and marmalade. She always cooks during the day and usually has a meal with meat or chicken plus vegetables and a lot of potatoes. In the evening, she eats banana sandwiches and can eat eight to ten slices of bread. She eats very little fruit and no sweets or cakes and drinks up to twelve cups of tea a day.

OBSERVATIONS

Jane's posture is very poor, with rounded, tense shoulders — she is quite stiff and finds it difficult to move quickly. She looks very pale and is very shaky. Her hair is in poor condition. Once she starts talking she can't stop, but she speaks in a very quiet voice. Her breath is very shallow and fast. She takes three mild tranquilizers a day.

TREATMENT

On this first visit, Jane was too distressed to have any in-depth shiatsu treatment.

I laid her down on the floor and encouraged her to start to breathe into her lower abdomen, which was not easy as her chest was so tense and her lower abdomen sore. After some minutes she started to relax and her breathing became easier. She sighed and yawned a lot. I encouraged her to tense and relax different muscles and she began to recognize how tense she was. I did a little shiatsu on her neck and shoulders.

ADVICE

- ten minutes of long, slow, deep breaths each day
- lie down and tense and relax different muscles in turn
- cut down on bread
- eat more fruit
- cut down on potatoes and try rice instead
- return in a week

Jane was much brighter after the session and more relaxed and at ease. She knew that she had gotten into a stressful state and arranged for someone to pick her up.

SECOND VISIT

Jane said that she felt well able to cope with life for two days following her first treatment and she appeared to have more confidence and openness on this visit. She had been practicing her breathing exercises and relaxation each day and her breathing had improved. Jane also looked brighter and made more of an effort about her appearance.

DIAGNOSIS

She lay down on the floor with greater ease than on the first occasion. I did a *hara* diagnosis and found that her kidney energy was very *kyo*; this was reflected in her anxiety, rest-lessness, lack of will to do anything, and her fear and appre-hension. Her spleen area was very *jitsu*. This can show in the body in obesity, poor strength, thinking too much and excessive concern for others. There was also a tightness and sense of blockage in the small intestine area.

TREATMENT

I first did some more relaxation exercises with Jane. Then, as she lay on her front, I did some shiatsu on the kidney and bladder meridians. Her lower back felt very weak and un-supported and I did some stretches and holding here to encourage energy to the area. I paid particular attention to kidney 1 point on the sole of the foot, which was very sore. I then did some stretches for the spleen meridian and worked thumbing up the meridian, where there was a lot of tender-ness. Jane almost fell asleep during the treatment.

ADVICE

- exercises to loosen her shoulders and to strengthen her lower back
- have more root vegetables in soups and stews, which will help to balance the spleen energy
- reduce tea intake, since this encourages stress in the body
- practice the lower back exercises twice a day to help strengthen the kidney area
- focus on the tendency to worry, try to name the worry and then pause and try to think of something else
- to return in a week

THIRD VISIT

Jane had made an effort to follow the recommendations. Her abdomen was no longer bloated, probably due to decreasing her bread intake to two slices a day and the fact that she is doing regular relaxation exercises and walking each day. Her color had improved and her posture was more erect.

Diagnosis

On *hara* diagnosis, her kidney energy was still very low but her spleen seemed less *jitsu*. Jane said that she was worrying less, felt physically much better and mentally had regained strength she had forgotten she had. She is going out and about more and wants to join a yoga class.

Advice

• return in a week

Fourth Visit

Jane returned and was radiant in comparison to how she has been. She felt that she was slowly returning to her old self. She decided to give up meat altogether and asked for information on vegetarian cooking classes. She was sleeping much better and also wanted to stop taking her tranquilizers.

Diagnosis

In *hara* diagnosis Jane's energy was much more balanced and the deficiency in her kidney *ki* was less remarkable. Her overall *ki* was stronger and there was more of a feeling of life from her.

Outcome

Over the following few months, Jane came for a shiatsu treatment every two weeks. In general, her attitude became more positive and she began to see that it was unnecessary to put so much energy into worrying about other people's problems. She also noticed her own health improving and it was no longer such a worry to her.

After a year, Jane was no longer taking tranquilizers. She still had an underlying fear of blindness and cancer, but was not as driven by these fears. At about this time, Jane had to go for an annual eye examination, the results of which were that she had to have an operation to prevent cataracts — news Jane coped with remarkably well. Following the operation she did not have the anxious time that she thought she might.

Jane has had a series of family crises over the last year and has remained calm and centered. She practices meditation daily and does some stretching exercises and walking. She no longer eats meat and cooks herself a vegetarian meal each day. When she gets low or anxious, she comes in for a few sessions and this so far has prevented her from going back into the depression and anxiety of earlier years.

CASE TWO: SIMON

Simon is a twenty-three-year-old man who lives at home with his mother and works in an office. He decided to try shiatsu because he had heard that it was good for head-aches. He had been to a number of doctors and specialists who were unable to find any relief for his symptoms.

REASON FOR VISIT

Simon has had a pain in his head and neck for a year and is constantly worried about it. He gets a lot of migraine-type headaches and blurring of vision. He has had his eyes tested and has been to specialists who have tested him for various potential problems — all the results have been negative. He has very sensitive skin and his face flares up with any change of temperature, or stress. Simon has a lot of fear and apprehension about his condition and finds communication difficult.

SIMON'S DIET

Oatmeal with milk and sugar for breakfast, followed by toast and butter and two cups of tea. During the morning he has a scone and butter and more tea. He goes home for lunch and has a full meal of meat, fresh vegetables and potatoes or rice. He eats red meat four times a week and chicken three times. He always has a dessert, with cream and sugar on it. In the evening, he usually has toast and cheese or a cheese sandwich or a salad, followed by tea and cookies. Simon drinks eight to ten cups of tea a day, does not smoke and does not drink much alcohol.

OBSERVATIONS

Simon is shy and withdrawn and has no interest in anything. He has very red, blotchy skin. He has dark circles around his eyes and is constantly blinking. Simon is thin and seems to have low energy. Close to tears, he has a lot of little nervous twitches.

HARA DIAGNOSIS

His kidney area *kyo* and felt very depleted — fears, phobias and lack of motivation are all associated with kidney imbalance. Triple heater area *jitsu*; difficulty in regulating body temperature, tension in the neck and shoulders and poor social skills are all a reflection of triple heater imbalance.

TREATMENT

I gave Simon breathing and relaxation exercises and neck and shoulder shiatsu, only a little, as his neck — which had very poor flexibility — was so sensitive. I tonified the *kyo* kidney meridian, which was also very sensitive. I worked on the triple heater meridian and did some stretches for the neck and shoulders.

The result was that Simon relaxed somewhat and then became really shivery at the end of the treatment; he was shaking all over and quite fearful. I covered him in blankets and he stopped shaking and felt better, though a little nauseous. I explained that when the body starts to let go of tension there can be a drop in temperature.

ADVICE

- daily relaxation exercise, tensing and relaxing all the muscle groups in turn

- neck rotations and neck stretches

- eliminate dairy foods for a month and then review

- decrease tea intake to three cups a day

- decrease red meat and have fish in its place

- return in a week

SECOND VISIT

Simon said that he had relief from his symptoms for three days, which he could not believe. His breathing had improved and eyes did not seem as strained. He found it difficult to give up tea, but said that he had not had a migraine all week, though some discomfort in his head returned after three days.

TREATMENT

I did some work on Simon's neck and shoulders and he was more relaxed and less fearful. The lung meridian was *kyo* today — I tonified it and also worked on the *kyo* kidney meridian. Simon responded well to some simple stretches and yawned a lot when I was finished. He felt cold following the treatment, but not as bad as last week.

ADVICE

- continue as before

- pay more attention to how he tenses up in difficult situations

- return in two weeks

THIRD VISIT

Again Simon had relief for three days following the shiatsu, which he was delighted about. On the fourth day he started to experience discomfort in the back of his head and neck. Simon has completely given up tea and does not miss it. He eats almost no dairy foods and has red meat only once a week. He has had no migraine headaches since the first treatment and his face does not flare up quite so much these days.

TREATMENT

I worked a lot on his neck and shoulders on this visit since they were less sensitive. I also did some *hara* shiatsu. Simon relaxed, his breathing slowed down a lot and became very deep. He again yawned a great deal. His kidney meridian was not so *kyo*. I worked on this and the triple heater, which again was *jitsu*.

ADVICE

- return in two weeks

FOURTH VISIT

He had relief from his symptoms for almost a week and felt full of energy and life — he was doing things that he had not done for years. Simon's eyes are not as strained and he is not blinking as much as before. His energy seemed more vibrant and he had opened up somewhat.

TREATMENT

The kidney is still the most *kyo* area but not as remarkable as on the first visits. I did some more shiatsu on him.

ADVICE

- go to a yoga class
- continue with his own relaxation

OUTCOME

Simon continued to have shiatsu once a month for a year and his condition had really improved by the end of this time. He attended yoga classes, joined a gym and a hill walking club and began to have an active social life again. He also became very interested in alternative therapies. He isolated his head discomfort to the times when he is under extreme pressure. He is more aware that he should not get into these situations, and he also has an understanding of how to manage his stress level.

CASE THREE: NAOMI

Naomi is a thirty-three-year-old woman who is married with a two-year-old child. She wanted to try some alternative treatment for recurrent chest infections and pain in her chest. Other things also came to light over the weeks of treatment.

MEDICAL HISTORY

Naomi had post-partum depression after the birth of her baby.

NAOMI'S DIET

Very meat-centered, with a lot of convenience foods — she eats a lot of refined rather than fresh foods. She has a weakness for cheese, eats very little fruit and has six to eight caffeine drinks daily. Naomi does not sit down to eat slowly, but mostly eats on the run.

FIRST VISIT

Naomi was complaining of chest infections recurring for the last year. She has had many courses of antibiotics and her energy is very low. She has a lot of mood swings and gets very little support from her husband, who minds their child while she works full time. She has almost no time to herself and feels uncomfortable if she has nothing to do.

OBSERVATIONS

Naomi has poor posture, rounded shoulders and a pale/ yellowish complexion. The top half of her body looks life-less and weak and the bottom half sluggish. Her breathing is very shallow. She speaks very fast, with a whine in her voice, and complains a lot. She is close to tears much of the time. She appears to be a perfectionist and creates a lot of stress for herself by having to have the house tidy all the time.

HARA DIAGNOSIS

Liver felt *jitsu* — tense, with the energy stagnant. *Jitsu* liver is associated with unresolved anger, control and exhaustion due to excessive drive. The lung area felt *kyo* with a sense of the energy lacking, which is reflected in Naomi's inability to create space for herself, her chest problems plus her melancholy and negative attitude.

TREATMENT

I showed Naomi how to breathe in a more efficient way from her lower abdomen and went through a relaxation exercise with her. I used a lot of stretches during the treatment to encourage energy flow. I energized the *kyo* lung meridian and worked on its pair, the large intestine, which felt sluggish — Naomi said that she is frequently constipated. While I was working on the lung, she yawned a lot and began to let go and relax. While she was lying in the prone position, I used some scattering techniques to relax the tense liver area in the mid-back. I also worked on the liver meridian in the legs and did some stretches. I then proceeded with a more general shiatsu treatment to encourage relaxation.

The result was that Naomi felt a lot more relaxed and was better able to communicate and express herself. She was pleased that someone was really listening to her. She then spoke about her anger about having to go to work rather than looking after her child. The pain in her chest was considerably better by the end of the session and her breathing had noticeably improved.

ADVICE

- spend at least ten minutes a day concentrating on breathing slowly while lying on the floor with one hand on the lower abdomen, feeling it rise and fall with the in- and out-breath

- notice how difficult this simple exercise is

- become conscious of breathing and the events that make the breath change

- lie on the back on a pile of cushions each evening with arms extended over head; stay in this position for some minutes, feeling the chest opening up

- do the lung and large intestine meridian stretch regularly during the day

- talk more with her husband instead of building up resentment

- no dairy foods for a month because they cause mucus congestion

- no coffee or tea for a month

- more fresh foods and less packet/refined foods

- hot cereal each morning

- fresh fruit during the day instead of cookies and cakes

- less red meat and more fish and green vegetables — these are lighter and more easily digested

- eat slowly and mindfully, noticing how often the food is finished before you have started to pay attention

- return in two weeks.

SECOND VISIT

Naomi returned looking brighter and more alive. The most obvious change was in the tone of her voice — it was lighter. She was more comfortable looking at me when speaking. Her cough had completely cleared up. She was less tired, though still did not have much surplus energy.

She is following the recommendations given.

DIAGNOSIS

On this visit, Naomi's *kyo* lung diagnosis was similar though not quite as remarkable as on the first visit. Her large intestine meridian felt more balanced and her constipation had improved. Although still stressed, she had more of an awareness of how she is creating this condition for herself.

TREATMENT

This consisted of a lot of holding to draw energy to the upper body, some stretching and specific work on the lung and large intestine meridians. Her neck and shoulders were very tense and I did some work on these.

OUTCOME

Naomi came regularly for treatment for a few months and slowly her condition improved. The most notable changes were the lack of chest infections and the brighter outlook that she adopted. Her bowel habits became regular. She started yoga classes and found them useful.

It is now some years since Naomi first came for treatment. She has two more children and is coping well. She is still prone to depression and a feeling that she cannot cope and needs more support, but a shiatsu treatment always makes her feel more positive and better able to manage.

She has stayed off dairy foods as much as possible and has almost given up red meat. What Naomi needed more than anything was to take time out for herself, to slow down and make space to reflect on the things that create discomfort for her. Coming for regular treatment was a positive step in recognizing her needs and getting some nourishing/supportive treatment.

HELPFUL ADDRESSES

In order to find a professional practitioner, you can contact the appropriate country's governing body of shiatsu. Most countries with a number of shiatsu schools will have a list of professionally qualified practitioners. There are also many individuals who do not register with a society for official recognition and are very fine practitioners — word of mouth is a good way to find the right practitioner for you.

American Oriental Bodywork
   Therapy Association (AOBTA)
Laurel Oak and Corporate Center, Suite 408
1010 Haddonfield–Berlin Road
Voorhees, NJ 08043
Tel.: 609-782-1616
Fax: 609-782-1653

RECOMMENDED READING

Hanh, Thich Nhat, *The Long Road Turns to Joy: A Guide to Walking Meditation*. Parallax Press, 1996.

Hanh, Thich Nhat, *Miracle of Mindfulness: A Manual on Meditation*. Beacon Press, 1996.

Kornfield, Jack, *A Path with Heart: A Guide through the Perils and Promises of Spiritual Life*. Bantam Doubleday Dell Publishing, 1993.

Lundberg, Paul, *The Book of Shiatsu*. Simon & Schuster, 1992.

Masunaga, Shizuto, *Zen Shiatsu: How to Harmonize Yin and Yang for Better Health*. Japan Publications, 1977.

Ohashi, Wataru, *Do-It-Yourself Shiatsu: How to Perform the Ancient Japanese Art of "Acupuncture Without Needles."* Arkana, 1992.

Pitchford, P., *Healing with Wholefoods; Oriental Traditions and Modern Nutrition*, Rev. ed. North Atlantic Books, 1993.

Suzuki, Shunryu, *Zen Mind, Beginner's Mind*. Weatherhill, 1988.

Tsu, Lao, *Tao Te Ching*. Vintage Books, 1997.

Weil, Andrew, *Spontaneous Healing*. Knopf, 1995.

The Yellow Emperor's Classic of Internal Medicine. University of California Press, 1966.

INDEX

NOTES

NOTES

NOTES

NOTES

ULYSSES PRESS HEALTH BOOKS

DISCOVER HANDBOOKS

Easy to follow and authoritative, *Discover Handbooks* reveal an array of alternative therapies from around the world and demonstrate how to incorporate them into a program of good health.

Each book opens with information on the history and principles of the particular technique, then presents practical and straightforward guidance on ways in which it can be applied. Offering the tools needed to achieve and maintain an optimal state of health, the approach is one of personal improvement and self-reliance. Each of the books features: an introduction to the discipline; an explanation of its philosophy; step-by-step guide to its implementation; clear diagrams and charts; and case studies.

DISCOVER AYURVEDA
ISBN 1-56975-081-5, 128 pp, $8.95

DISCOVER COLOR THERAPY
ISBN 1-56975-093-9, 144 pp, $8.95

DISCOVER ESSENTIAL OILS
ISBN 1-56975-080-7, 128 pp, $8.95

DISCOVER FLOWER ESSENCES
ISBN 1-56975-099-8, 120 pp, $8.95

DISCOVER MEDITATION
ISBN 1-56975-113-7, 144 pp, $8.95

DISCOVER NUTRITIONAL THERAPY
ISBN 1-56975-135-8, 120 pp, $8.95

DISCOVER OSTEOPATHY
ISBN 1-56975-115-3, 132 pp, $8.95

DISCOVER REFLEXOLOGY
ISBN 1-56975-112-9, 132 pp, $8.95

DISCOVER SHIATSU
ISBN 1-56975-082-3, 128 pp, $8.95

A Natural Approach Books

Written in a friendly, nontechnical style, *A Natural Approach* books address specific health issues and show you how to take an active part in your own treatment. Whether you suffer from panic attacks, endometriosis or depression, each book will provide you with a thorough understanding of your condition and detail organic solutions that offer immediate relief for your symptoms and effectively remedy their underlying causes.

Believing that disease is more than a combination of symptoms, these books offer integrated mind/body programs that take a positive, preventative approach. Since traditional drug therapy is not always the best solution (and can sometimes be the problem), these guides show how to use alternative treatments to supplement or replace conventional medicine.

ANXIETY & DEPRESSION
ISBN 1-56975-118-8, 144 pp, $9.95

ENDOMETRIOSIS
ISBN 1-56975-088-2, 120 pp, $8.95

FREE YOURSELF FROM TRANQUILIZERS
& SLEEPING PILLS
ISBN 1-56975-074-2, 192 pp, $9.95

IRRITABLE BLADDER & INCONTINENCE
ISBN 1-56975-089-0, 108 pp, $8.95

IRRITABLE BOWEL SYNDROME
ISBN 1-56975-030-0, 240 pp, $11.95

MIGRAINES
ISBN 1-56975-140-4, 156 pp, $8.95

PANIC ATTACKS
ISBN 1-56975-045-9, 148 pp, $8.95

The Natural Healer Books

As home remedies and alternative treatments become increasingly accepted into the medical mainstream, people want information—not just hype and unproven claims—about the remedies they see in health food stores. *The Natural Healer* books detail how these natural remedies have been used throughout history and how to safely incorporate them into an overall plan for maintaining good health.

CIDER VINEGAR
ISBN 1-56975-141-2, 120 pp, $8.95

GARLIC
ISBN 1-56975-097-1, 120 pp, $8.95

THE ANCIENT AND
HEALING ARTS BOOKS

The Ancient and Healing Arts books recount the development of healing art forms that have been used for thousands of years. Beautifully illustrated with full color on every page, they discuss the benefits of these time-honored techniques and offer detailed instructions on their use.

THE ANCIENT AND HEALING ART OF
AROMATHERAPY
ISBN 1-56975-094-7, 96 pp, $14.95

THE ANCIENT AND HEALING ART OF
CHINESE HERBALISM
ISBN 1-56975-139-0, 96 pp, $14.95

OTHER HEALTH TITLES

THE BOOK OF KOMBUCHA
ISBN 1-56975-049-1, 160 pp, $11.95
Explains the benefits of and addresses concerns about Kombucha, the widely used Chinese "tea mushroom."

HEPATITIS C: A PERSONAL GUIDE TO GOOD HEALTH
ISBN 1-56975-091-2, 172 pp, $12.95
Identifies the causes and symptoms of hepatitis C and presents conventional and alternative treatments for coping with the disease.

KNOW YOUR BODY: THE ATLAS OF ANATOMY
ISBN 1-56975-021-1, 160 pp, $12.95
Presents a full-color guide to the structure of the human body.

MOOD FOODS
ISBN 1-56975-023-8, 192 pp, $9.95
Shows how the foods you eat influence your emotions and behavior.

YOUR NATURAL PREGNANCY: A GUIDE TO COMPLEMENTARY THERAPIES
ISBN 1-56975-059-9, 240 pp, $16.95
Details alternative therapies ranging from aromatherapy to yoga that can benefit pregnant women.

To order these books call 800-377-2542, fax 510-601-8307 or write to Ulysses Press, P.O. Box 3440, Berkeley, CA 94703-3440. All retail orders are shipped free of charge. California residents must include sales tax. Allow two to three weeks for delivery.

Catherine Sutton runs a private shiatsu clinic in Dublin, Ireland.